Nerve Block
for Common Pain

Richard Cytowic

Nerve Block
for Common Pain

With 7 Illustrations

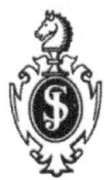

Springer-Verlag
New York Berlin Heidelberg
London Paris Tokyo Hong Kong

Richard Cytowic, M.D.
Capitol Neurology
1611 Connecticut Avenue N.W.
Washington, D.C. 20009-1033
USA

Library of Congress Cataloging-in-Publication Data
Cytowic, Richard E.
    Nerve block for common pain / Richard Cytowic.
        p.   cm.
    Includes bibliographical references.
    ISBN-13:978-0-387-97147-6
    1. Pain—Treatment.   2. Nerve block.   I. Title.
RB127.C98   1990
616'.0472—dc20   89-21912

Printed on acid-free paper.

Typeset by David E. Seham Associates, Inc., Metuchen, New Jersey.

9 8 7 6 5 4 3 2 1

ISBN-13:978-0-387-97147-6   e-ISBN-13:978-1-4613-8950-7
DOI: 10.1007/978-1-4613-8950-7

Contents

1 —
Introduction

Background

The treatment of pain cuts across all specialties. While some will take a far greater interest in the treatment of pain than others, every physician must have some reasonable skill in its treatment. This handbook has two objectives. First, it reminds the physician of some options in treating pain, whether he uses them himself or refers patients to specialists. More importantly, however, it emphasizes an option that is extremely effective but underutilized, and which is also well within the skill of most physicians: nerve block.

Like anyone else, physicians are creatures of habit. We develop our own patterns of medical practice and soon establish psychological boundaries between what we feel comfortable and competent doing and what we consider beyond our expertise. Historically, training in nerve block seems to be limited to anesthesiologists and neurosurgeons, sometimes including neurologists. It is a technique, however, that can well be used by any physician. Injection blockade is both safe and effective for a number of very common pain syndromes. This handbook focuses on a small number of myofascial and neuritic pain syndromes that the busy practitioner will see repeatedly.

In the face of daily decisions and given the choice between the familiar and unfamiliar, frontline doctors will tend to do the familiar. The familiar, unfortunately, is likely to be a hodgepodge and often ineffective, most often dispensing oral analgesics and antiinflammatories. A common reason for treatment failure is that neither medical school nor residency provides any real education about treating pain, and only a minority of physicians have a well-thought-out plan or treatment algorithm for pain.

The utilization of nerve block varies considerably, even in specialized pain clinics. The specialty of the clinic director accounts for this difference. Clinics directed by anesthesiologists are *seven times* more likely to use nerve blocks than those directed by other specialists. The nonsurgical specialist who was not trained in the performance of nerve block may be reluctant to use them when there are other treatments to choose from. By virtue of familiarity, anesthesiologists are likely to view nerve blocks as more benign (Khoury and Varga, 1988).

Because this handbook is not about pain but about one type of pain relief, the focus must stay on nerve block. But precisely because there is so little systematic education about pain, I will necessarily review topics such as placebos, differences between acute and chronic pain, compensation, litigation, and malingering. The purpose of even discussing such topics is to clarify some very common misconceptions, and cannot be a comprehensive review. Suggested reading and references will help direct the interested reader to more thorough presentations.

Considerably past World War II, various neural blockades were the primary means of diagnosis and therapy for pain. Despite hundreds of modern papers on pain and the development of a few multidisciplinary pain centers in the United States, the attention to pain by most physicians was nil until the early 1970s, when a number of factors converged (Bonica, 1953, 1988). One was the Melzack–Wall (1966) Gate Theory of pain, which aroused worldwide curiosity about the mechanism and efficacy of acupuncture for both pain relief and surgical anesthesia. Another was the founding of the International Association for the Study of Pain in 1974, with the subsequent publication of its journal *Pain*.

Today, there are more alternatives in treating pain, and nerve block no longer occupies the position it once did. It is still, however, a prime choice. Nerve block is effective in some patients who do not receive adequate relief from drugs; some patients are able to stop oral medication for long periods after nerve block (Cousins, 1988). Pain relief from nerve block lasts far longer than the mere pharmacologic action of the drug injected. Sometimes a block, or series of blocks, can relieve pain permanently.

Hyperstimulation Analgesia

One of the oldest methods of pain relief is hyperstimulation analgesia produced by dry-needling myofascial trigger points, acupuncture, intense heat or cold, or chemical irritation of the skin. A brief painful stimulus may relieve chronic pain for long periods, sometimes permanently. According to gate theory, we conceive that pain is relieved by "closing the gate" by central biasing and by disrupting neural feedback loops responsible for the "memory" of pain. Hyperstimulation or anesthetic injection restores normal function and prevents recurrence of neural feedback. Clinical experience shows that *modulation of sensory inputs* by various techniques reduces pain much more than by surgically cutting sensory pathways. Worse yet, pain is likely to return after surgical ablation.

Melzack (1981) reviewed the relationship of myofascial trigger points to acupuncture and hyperstimulation analgesia. Trigger points often overlie classical acupuncture points. The success of hyperstimulation analgesia is explained by gate theory, and is represented in folk medicine by counterirritation treatments such as mustard plasters, ice packs, cupping, and blistering of the skin. Acupuncture is viewed similarly in terms of hyperstimulation.

A number of medical and social factors are known to decrease the success of nerve block in relieving chronic pain (Abram, Anderson & Maitre-D'Cruze, 1981). Some of the most important are long duration of pain, rating the pain as severe, and heavy analgesic use. Perhaps, then, the use of nerve block in the *acute* stage would prevent these consequences from ever developing.

This handbook emphasizes nerve block in the treatment of pain. We next review the general principles of nerve block and then briefly discuss some areas of pain treatment that perpetrate many misconceptions.

General Principles of Nerve Block

Table 1.1 capsulizes the benefits of nerve block (Bonica, 1988). Not only does neural blockade interrupt pain input at

TABLE 1.1. General principles of nerve block.[a]

Nerve block is *one* tool in multidisciplinary approach
Interruption of pain at or near its source
Interruption of abnormal reflexes (eg., muscle spasm) and vicious
     cycles
Sympathetic block eliminates sympathetic hyperactivity that
     contributes to pathophysiology of pain
Sympathetic block improves blood flow
Attention to physical aspect of pain may gain patient cooperation
     in exploring psychological issues
Nerve block may enhance patient–doctor relationship and be useful
     in overall rehabilitation strategy

[a]From Bonica, J. J. 1988. Neural blockade in the multidisciplinary pain clinic. In: Cousins, M. J., Bridenbaugh, P. O., eds. Neural Blockade, 2nd Ed. Copyright 1988 by Lippincott. Reprinted with permission.

its source, but it also interrupts the afferent limb of a vicious feedback loop believed to contribute to chronic pain syndrome. This may be one reason why pain relief lasts far longer than the pharmacologic action of the drug. Relief may sometimes last for days or weeks. Based on ideas from hyperstimulation analgesia, Melzack (1973) proposed that interrupting the sensory input stopped the feedback loops in spinal cord and brain. This reflex activity involves muscle spasm, changes in blood flow with tissue ischemia, release of active substances in interstitial tissues, and a host of cognitive and emotional changes as well.

Similarly, sympathetic blockade can interrupt the sympathetic hyperactivity seen with pain and also bring about changes in tissue blood flow. Pharmacologic properties of injected anesthetics are exploited, with low concentrations achieving selective blockade of unmyelinated C and B preganglionic fibers, and the small myelinated A delta pain fibers. Such a "differential block" produces minimal change in motor function.

Although nerve block is only one tool the physician can

use in a multidisciplinary approach to pain, it relates to other choices as well as psychological issues relevant to the individual patient. For example, if patients are reluctant to consider that their pain may have emotional factors, the initial focus on a physical intervention such as nerve block may release them to explore psychological issues.

Misconceptions and Management of Chronic Pain

My intention in mentioning topics such as placebo, fear of narcotic abuse, compensation, and others discussed here is to point out the widespread misconceptions about these sensitive matters. Such misconceptions lead to errors in the management of patients even when we emphasize only one treatment, which in our case is nerve block. While the topics themselves are complex, a short treatment of each will suffice to focus us on the overall attitude necessary in treating pain appropriately with any modality. Differences between acute and chronic pain are highlighted (Reuler, Girard & Nardone, 1980).

Placebos

Placebo comes from the Latin, meaning "I will please." A placebo is any therapeutic procedure given deliberately to have an effect, or that unintentionally has an effect, but which is objectively without specific activity for the condition being treated.

In the 1950s, Beecher (1955) showed that 35% of patients with organic pain obtained significant relief with a placebo. Later studies (Evans, 1974) showed that the effective index—that is, the amount of pain relief from placebo versus a specific analgesic—is a constant 0.55! In other words, the effectiveness of the placebo is directly proportional to the effectiveness of the active drug to which it is compared. A placebo will therefore be 50% as effective as morphine when compared to morphine and 50% as effective as aspirin when compared to aspirin. It seems likely that the endogenous endorphin system is responsible for placebo analgesia (Levine, Gordon & Fields, 1978), rather than such analgesia resulting from suggestibility or susceptibility to hypnosis. Indeed, the apparent mechanisms of placebo and narcotic analgesia appear to be similar: tolerance develops over long periods and withdrawal symptoms appear when the placebo is abruptly withheld. The placebo response can also be blocked by the narcotic antagonist naloxone, a feature few people realize.

There is considerable misunderstanding about the placebo effect. It is precisely the difficult and demanding patient who is *least likely* to respond to placebo compared to one who is well liked. A study of nursing and house staff showed that the majority grossly underestimated the percentage of patients who do respond to placebo. Sixty percent of physicians used placebos to "prove" whether the pain was "real," and 75% used them in acquiescing to nursing complaints about problem patients. A positive response to placebo was actually misinterpreted as proving that there was, in fact, no organic basis for the patient's pain (Goodwin, Goodwin & Vogel, 1979).

In contrast to this negative attitude, it is precisely an enthusiastic and expectant attitude that is critical to a positive placebo effect (Egbert, Battit, Welch & Bartlett, 1964). The 50% effectiveness seen in double-blind placebo trials suggests that even though the double blind is maintained, the therapist's enthusiasm is conveyed to the patient. Such results suggest that the overall effect of a real analgesic can be augmented by the manner in which its effectiveness is presented.

Other interesting and counterintuitive features of the placebo is that it is more effective for severe than mild pain; more effective in patients with greater stress and anxiety; and more effective in patients who are constitutionally anxious (trait anxiety) rather than just being anxious about their current circumstance (state anxiety). Moreover, two placebo pills work better than one; larger pills are better than small ones; injections are superior to pills; and potency increases when the physician suggests that a powerful pain-killer is being administered (Melzak, 1988).

The point is that a positive placebo response does not prove that the pain is "in the patient's head." Rather, it proves that the patient indeed perceives pain and is suffering. When treating pain with nerve block, the physician can and should deliberately invoke an adjuvant placebo response by being enthusiastic and expectant about its effectiveness. The patient will already have tried many treatments that have failed; the hope provided by an expectant and congenial physician–patient relationship should not be underestimated.

Acute Versus Chronic Pain

The division of pain into acute and chronic is not at all arbitrary, but is based on an increased understanding that the central modulation of acute and chronic pain differs as does its treatment and response.

While acute pain often has objective evidence—a clear temporal pattern of onset, objective physical signs, and autonomic hyperactivity—chronic pain does not. In chronic pain one finds adaptation of autonomic signs and marked changes in personality, lifestyle, and functional capacity (Foley, 1985; Sternbach, 1974). In addition to physical pain, patients must also handle emotional, social, bureaucratic, financial, and spiritual pain–Saunders (1967) has called this "total pain."

But what is pain? New knowledge has made it clear that pain is not just a simple sensory phenomenon but a most complex, multidimensional human experience caused by a surprising variety of physiological, psychological, and environmental factors.

The International Association for the Study of Pain calls it "an unpleasant sensory and emotional experience associated with actual or potential tissue damage or described in terms of such damage (Merskey, 1986)." Note the stress on emotional factors. But there is a caveat with this: It is all too easy to place patients in either/or categories wanting, on one hand, to "fix the problem" without taking a small amount of time to understand the patient's subjective experience or how the pain affects his daily life, while on the other summarily dismissing patients with few physical findings as "functional" and sending them off to the psychiatrist.

Obviously, a balance is necessary. The management of pain does not involve becoming a technical expert at inserting needles. The physician must have adequate knowledge of various pain syndromes and the usefulness, limitations, and complications of various modalities available for each syndrome. Rather than thinking that nerve block is an esoteric procedure to be done only by a technical consultant, the treating physician has much to offer in a holistic way when he is able to perform nerve block as one of the treatment options.

By any definition pain is a symptom of disease. Is it therefore justifiable to treat it as a separate entity? It would have been a grand mistake, for example, if the focus in infectious diseases had been on the fevers which many of them cause. But even in this subspecialty, which we understand in terms of the etiological infectious agent, the study of the symptomatic fever did in fact make a difference. It led to the separation of typhus from typhoid fever and tertian from quartan malaria. By analogy, the study of pain as a separate entity is quite justified in that it leads back to an understanding of the mechanism of pain. This feedback is sorely needed, because the mechanism of most pain syndromes is unknown, even in such conditions as postherpetic or occipital neuralgia in which the ultimate cause is known but the mechanism is lacking.

A moment's reflection will show that the oft-quoted maxim that pain is subjective is a needless disparagement. To say that the subjective experience of pain cannot be measured really begs the question. The real issue is not how measures are obtained but how reliable and valid they are. Apparently objective tests such as blood chemistries are subject to large errors, as much as 20%. It is delusion to assume that such tests, which do not involve introspective self-reporting, are more accurate than human observation or patient self-reporting. The diagnosis of specific pain is made by the characteristic history of quality, location, aggravating factors, and so forth. The word diagnosis means "through knowledge," not through machines or tests. The knowledge here, of course, is the physician's knowledge.

So, even though there may be limited objective signs to confirm the presence or severity of the patient's pain, physician and patient are best served if the physician accepts the patient's report at face value. Reliability, not objectivity, is the important issue.

There are important differences between acute and chronic pain. In acute pain, the nervous system is usually intact; the pain is caused by an identifiable trauma, surgery, or medical illness. Facial grimacing is common, and patients know that the end is in sight because the pain usually stops when their condition resolves. Increased autonomic activity such as hypertension, tachycardia, diaphoresis, muscle spasm, and changes in gastrointestinal secretion and motility and in venous stasis are seen. These are mediated through segmental and suprasegmental reflexes.

Chronic pain is arbitrarily defined as lasting past the time of healing, 3 months or more. Sympathetic-adrenal responses habituate, and vegetative ones emerge. The patient's capacity for physical, mental, and social coping also become exhausted, and a subdued facial expression often leads to the erroneous impression that such patients cannot be experiencing any pain. These features of chronic, unrelieved pain may be rapidly reversed if the pain is stopped.

Characteristics of Patients with Chronic Pain

Preconceptions and truisms abound regarding chronic pain patients despite numerous studies showing these to be false. A composite stereotype of such deadbeats is a blue-collar

TABLE 1.2. Problems reported by patients with chronic pain ($n = 165$).[a]

Problem	Men	Women	Total
Physical illness	56	47	103
Finances	41	32	73
Sex difficulties	38	14	52
Work situation	19	13	32
Children	10	13	23
Change in personality	7	9	16
Parents/in-laws	5	9	14
House & environment	4	6	10
Religion	5	0	5

[a]From Colvin, D. F. Bettinger, R. Knapp, R. Pawlicki, R. Zimmerman J. 1980. Characteristics of patients with chronic pain. South. Med. J. 73(8). Copyright 1980 by Southern Medical Association. Reprinted with permission.

worker, poorly educated, receiving workmen's compensation, and perhaps bringing litigation.

Colvin et al. (1980) reported on the characteristics of 300 such patients at the West Virginia University Pain Clinic. Patients were just as likely to be male as female, be a high-school graduate as not, to be between 40 and 60 years old, and unemployed and receiving compensation because of their pain. Fifty-two percent of their patients were high school graduates and 20% had further education, including 10% who graduated from college or professional school.

The three most frequent patient problems were physical illness, finances, and sexual difficulties (Table 1.2). Sexual difficulty was the only problem that was statistically different between men and women, men being more likely to report difficulty. Almost half of both sexes reported a big decline in libido, with only one in five patients remaining as sexually active as they were before the onset of their pain.

Patients with chronic pain appear to be quite fearful. One-third believed their pain was caused by something more serious than the doctor was telling them, while 50% thought they had not received an adequate explanation for their misery. An empirical assessment of pain beliefs (Williams & Thorn, 1989) showed that patients' own conceptualization of what pain is and means to them may be discordant with current scientific understanding and may adversely affect compliance with treatment. Self-blame, perception of pain as mysterious, and expectations about the duration of pain correlated positively with an increased perception of pain and decreased compliance.

Instead of yet another treatment failure, the physician can achieve a treatment success by accepting the patient's report at face value, recognizing that the absence of obvious agony is characteristic of chronic pain, and directly addressing the patient's fears, which are almost never spontaneously voiced.

Compensation, Litigation, Malingering, and Unemployment

Neurotic features are a consequence, not a cause, of pain. Unfortunately, applying the principles of the disease model forces one to pigeonhole pain patients into organic or psychogenic categories. Environment does indeed influence behavior, and organic lesions that produce pain will also, with time, produce emotional and psychological changes (Merskey & Boyd, 1978). Psychometric testing instruments such as the Minnesota Multiphasic Personality Inventory (MMPI) are not able to distinguish between organic and psychogenic pain. Both have increased scores on hypochondriasis and depression scales. The classification of patients into four types based on their MMPI profiles (hypochondriacal, reactively depressed, somaticizers, and manipulators) is empirically reproducible and rich in implications for behavioral treatment (Sternbach, 1974, 1976).

With no more authority than common sense that "everybody knows," much stock has been placed in compensation, litigation, and unemployment as being regular accompaniments of chronic pain if not pathognomonic for malingering. Well-constructed studies designed to objectively look at these factors, however, explode these myths as false. One of the confounds in analyzing these relationships is that chronic pain patients who are receiving compensation or who have litigation pending are, in fact, less likely to be working. Dworkin et al. (1985) showed that in multiple regression analysis only employment was a significant factor in predicting a good outcome. The analysis of both short- and long-term treatment response showed that patients who were working at the time of their initial evaluation had a better response to treatment than patients who were not working. The inconsistent results of studies examining relationships between compensation or litigation and treatment response could be explained by this confound of differences in the percentage of patients with compensation or litigation who are also employed.

Better results are obtained by forgetting about "compensation neurosis" and directing attention instead toward employment and *actively engaging the patient in his own treatment* (Weighill, 1983). In a study of back injury, the longer the patient was unemployed the less likelihood he would return to work (Beals & Hickman, 1972). Based on such results, at least one chronic pain program (Catchlove & Cohen, 1982) directed patients to return to work as part of their treatment. Significantly more patients did return to work when so instructed, and 90% of them were still working after an average follow-up of 9.6 months.

Most studies find few important differences when pain patients who are receiving compensation are compared to those who are not. Patients receiving compensation do not have a greater number of nonorganic signs and do not exhibit greater levels of psychological distress. A similar negative correlation holds for litigation. Chronic pain patients in litigation do not differ from those not litigating with respect to nonorganic signs, their description of pain or psychological distress, and various indicators of pain behavior (Peck,

Fordyce & Black, 1978; Dworkin et al., 1985). Mendelson (1982) showed that there is no evidence to support the truism that once settlement occurs patients quickly resume work. Kelley (1981) also showed this, as well as the fact that delaying settlement actually *increases the likelihood of never returning to work.* Average time from injury to settlement for his 170 subjects was 3.8 years for those not back at work before settlement, compared to 3.0 years for those who did return before settlement. Age and occupation influence the ability to return to work, with older patients and those in more dangerous occupations tending never to return. Similar relationships are seen in patients with chronic pain after concussion (Cytowic, Stump & Larned, 1988).

The point is that those who take the time to look will find that such patients manifest a wide variety of objective findings commensurate with injury to the central and peripheral nervous systems. Voltaire was more strident: The greater the ignorance, the greater the dogma. Ignorant dogma about "compensation neurosis" has been replaced by clear data showing that patients with or without compensation respond equally well to treatment, provided that treatment is adequate (Mendelson, 1984; Melzack, 1988).

But it is not ignorance alone that explains this professional bias. Kelly (1981; Kelly & Smith, 1981) suggested that organic "symptoms may be neurotically prolonged because of failure of the medical profession to recognize" them. Patient resentment is common, understandable, and "compounded when they meet disbelief from the medical profession and lawyers, a refusal to treat their symptoms, and a vague hint of moral disapproval."

It may surprise some to discover that physicians agree that malingering is a relatively infrequent condition, occurring in less than 5% of cases. Data from 105 specialists show that agreement increases with clinical symptoms reflecting exaggeration of pain and incongruous behavior (Leavitt & Sweet, 1986). Specialists who were high estimators of malingering placed great emphasis, incorrectly, on the fact that patients were on compensation or had seen an attorney.

Concordance of 70% or more on six separate clinical behaviors suggests that there is considerably more agreement among clinicians as to what to look for than had been previously appreciated. Exaggeration and incongruity were the two basic dimensions, and included the following items: overaction during exam, disablement disproportionate to objective findings, weakness to manual testing not seen in other activities, pain not following organic patterns, and endorsement of false symptom suggestions.

Nonetheless, even its low incidence makes malingering an important problem when the incidence of an illness is high. For example, in the United States alone, more than 8 million patients seek treatment for back pain yearly (Mayer, 1983). If 3% are malingering, there are 240,000 annual problem cases.

Behavioral Approaches to Pain

Behavioral approaches promote an increased sense of control by reducing feelings of helplessness and hopelessness commonly associated with chronic pain. They also break the vicious cycle of pain–anxiety–tension. Few controlled studies, however, compare their effectiveness with standard medical or surgical therapies. It is believed that these methods are helpful because they modulate the affective response to pain. Fifty percent of patients receive pain relief by hypnosis, for example, although there is no one single effective hypnotic procedure. Moreover, the analgesia induced by hypnosis is not mediated by the endogenous opiate system because it does not reverse by naloxone (Mayer & Price, 1976).

Negative behavioral approaches may be iatrogenic. A study of house officers (Charap, 1978) gives a classic example of iatrogenic operant conditioning, because house officers thought that dosage p.r.n. was ideal because it minimized tolerance, a false notion. Experimentally, anxiety influences pain perception. Great anxiety accompanies the anticipation of recurrent pain, increasing both the perception of the pain and the analgesic dose required. Because medication is repeatedly associated with relief from agony, a p.r.n. schedule provides reinforcement that leads to psychological dependence. These problems can be avoided by simply putting the patient on a regular schedule of medication. Moreover, it is much easier to treat moderate pain than severe pain. Stalwart types should be educated not to wait until they are in agony because then any treatment, including nerve block, will not be very effective.

Individual requirements for analgesia vary considerably. The optimum dosage is the least amount required, repeated often enough to produce the desired therapeutic effect. Lack of knowledge of the equivalent analgesic dose when changing from one drug to another is the most common cause of undermedication. Likewise, the plasma half-lives do not correlate well with duration of clinical pain relief.

Narcotic Analgesics and Fear of Analgesic Abuse

Traditionally, narcotic analgesics have been used to manage acute pain; these are not used in chronic pain for fear of physical or psychological dependence. Because both patients and physicians, and patients even more than their doctors, hold the misconception that physical dependence and psychological dependence (addiction) are synonymous, the use of narcotic analgesics in either acute or chronic pain remains inadequate. Suffice it to say that patient fear—of addiction, of perceived weakness, from cultural bias—and the physician's lack of pharmacologic knowledge continues to limit the effective and optimum use of narcotic analgesics (Marks & Sachar, 1973; Sriwatanakul et al., 1983). Although the situation should have changed with the discovery of the endorphin system, it has not. Lack of dissemination is the most probable reason.

The practitioner interested in the long-term use of oral narcotics for chronic pain should know that extensive experience from the hospice movement shows that patients indeed show tolerance and physical dependence, but that psychological dependence (addiction) is rare (Angell, 1982; Porter & Jick, 1980). The interested practitioner will wish to consult guidelines by the American Medical Association (McGivey & Crooks, 1984) and the American College of Physicians (1983) for drug therapy in chronic pain patients with advanced disease. See also Foley (1985) for a review and practical recommendations.

The treatment of cancer pain is beyond the scope and intent of this handbook (Foley, 1985; Twycross & Fairfield, 1982; Cousins, 1988). Clinical experiences suggests that patients with cancer pain are best treated with a multidisciplinary approach.

There is no perfect choice among analgesics or other treatments for pain. The practitioner will save himself much anxiety and recrimination if he remembers this. Rather, it is the physician's knowledge of pharmacologic properties that should direct his choice among a series of agents and lead to the most effective use of a drug. There are no poor or dangerous drugs; only poor and dangerous uses of them. All drugs, from aspirin to azathioprine, have side effects.

Summary

Nerve block is one tool in a multidisciplinary approach to pain. Chronic pain differs from acute pain in that there are far fewer objective signs; autonomic responses have adapted, emotional and psychological features have emerged, and the patient is worn out. Tried-and-true approaches often have failed, and the physician who hopes to make a successful intervention needs to provide hope, to convey an enthusiastic and expectant attitude, and to accept the patient's complaint initially at face value. Knowledge of compensation, litigation, narcotic use, and other charged issues will correctly inform his decisions. His attitude is confident rather than uncertain, and patients are encouraged to return to work or regular activities as soon as feasible and to also assume an active role in their own care. With this approach, the physician is ready to offer and effectively use nerve block.

Further Reading

For the physician who either has or develops a further interest in treatment of pain, the following references are recommended.

Diagnosis and Evaluation

Rudy, T.E., Turk, D.C., Brena, S.F. 1988. Differential utility of medical procedures in the assessment of chronic pain patients. Pain 34:53–60.

Williams, R.C. 1988. Toward a set of reliable and valid measures for chronic pain assessment and outcome research. Review article. Pain 35:239–251.

2 —
The Muscular Origin of Pain

The passage of time does not resolve myofascial pain, although the response to bupivacaine injection is immediate and complete. Myofascial trigger-point injection is the simplest, safest, and most frequent anesthetic block. This type of field anesthesia does not require great expertise and gives gratifying results in a wide variety of common pains.

Basic Concepts

Myofascial trigger-point pain has been described in the medical and dental literature for well over a century. A safe, reliable, and effective means of treatment by local procaine injection was described by Lange in Germany and Steindler in the United States in the early decades of this century (Kraus, 1970). In this country, the principal proponent of myofascial pain has been Janet Travell, who was White House physician to Presidents Kennedy and Johnson. She frequently injected President Kennedy's back, injured during the war. These injections were so successful in keeping the President mobile that few people realized how disabled he actually was by his orthopedic condition and his chronic pain.

Today, myofascial trigger points are defined as "hyperirritable spots, usually within a taut band of skeletal muscle or in the muscle's fascia that is painful on compression and can give rise to characteristic referred pain, tenderness, and autonomic phenomena" (Travell & Simons, 1983). Current practice uses bupivacaine to anesthetize these trigger points. Years of clinical experience has shown bupivacaine to be safe and effective when used appropriately.

It is characteristic that trigger-point bupivacaine injections provide pain relief and return of function (increased range of motion, resolution of muscle spasm, and decreased allodynia) far outlasting the pharmacologic action of local anesthesia and far in excess of any therapeutic benefit gained by saline injection or dry-needling (acupuncture). The mechanism for this is not clear. While some suggest there is an additional placebo response, one must realize that the therapeutic response of trigger-point injections is long lasting and often curative. The trigger-point concept has been difficult for physicians to accept because the precise neuroanatomy between the trigger point and pain perception is not understood. Nonetheless, motor unit potentials are recorded when the trigger point is palpated, and biopsy shows waxy degeneration of muscle fibers, fatty infiltration, and an increase in nuclei (Travell & Simons, 1983).

Although neither the exact pathogenesis of a trigger point nor the mechanism of its cure by injection has been clearly elucidated, the therapeutic effect of trigger-point injections does involve the endogenous opioid system, just as the analgesic effects of transcutaneous electrical stimulation and acupuncture do. All three treatments are reversible by naloxone (Fine, Melano & Hare, 1988).

The biologic half-life of the endogenous opioid peptides is relatively short—on the order of minutes. Thus, simply activating their synthesis or release could not adequately account for the lengthy analgesia produced by bupivacaine injections. By comparison to the mechanism of sympathetically maintained pain, some suggest that a reflex arc is established that has both central and peripheral components. A plausible candidate for the central component are the wide dynamic range (WDR) neurons in the spinal cord. These remain sensitized despite resolution of the original injury. There is then a decrease in the threshold of peripheral mechanoreceptors whose afferents converge on the WDR neurons, and increased rate of firing from the ascending projections from the WDR neurons, resulting in painful sensations (Fine, Melano & Hare, 1988; Roberts, 1986). More will be said in the discussion of reflex sympathetic dystrophy and sympathetically mediated pain in Chapter 5.

Location of Trigger Points

Myofascial structures refer pain in predictable patterns that do not follow a segmental distribution. The consistent location of trigger points as well as the pattern of referred pain eases diagnosis. The trigger point is a physical finding disclosed on examination. Myofascial pain is one of the most important causes of functional disability, stemming partially from its frequency. As Travell (1976) points out, "many physicians fail to recognize and treat them, but if these conditions are properly diagnosed and effectively treated, patients are spared prolonged disability."

Pain of muscular origin rarely leads the list of differential diagnoses, and skeletal muscles are almost never examined. This situation is unfortunate. Patient examination today is so dependent on machines that the manual examination of the body is a lost art. Current medical education is not sufficient in functional anatomy or kinesiology.

Patients, too, conceive of their pain in terms of concrete mechanisms, such as pinched nerves and arthritis, yet have difficulty believing that sudden stretching or overactivity of their muscles can lead to such persistent pain. True joint pain (arthritis) is quite characteristic; likewise, true radiculopathy is associated with neurological findings (areflexia, weakness, segmental sensory loss). Trigger-point pain has none of these features.

Skeletal muscle accounts for 40% of body weight. Any muscle can develop trigger points that cause pain and muscle spasm, although some locations are much more common that others (Figure 2.1). They do not hold fixed positions like classical acupuncture points, nor are they synonymous with motor points (which are found by electrical stimulation, not palpation). Little progress in understanding this condition has been made since muscle hardness and callouses, or "Muskelhärten" and "Muskelschwiele," were described by German authors at the end of the 18th century. Britons used the term myogelosis to describe the muscle's gelatinous firmness (Simons, 1975). Much confusion in understanding this painful condition arises from the variety of terms: muscular rheumatism, idiopathic myalgia, fibromyalgia, and fibrositis (McCain and Scudds, 1988). Emphasis on regional anatomy led to terms such as tennis elbow and housemaid's knee. These are just instances of a generic condition that

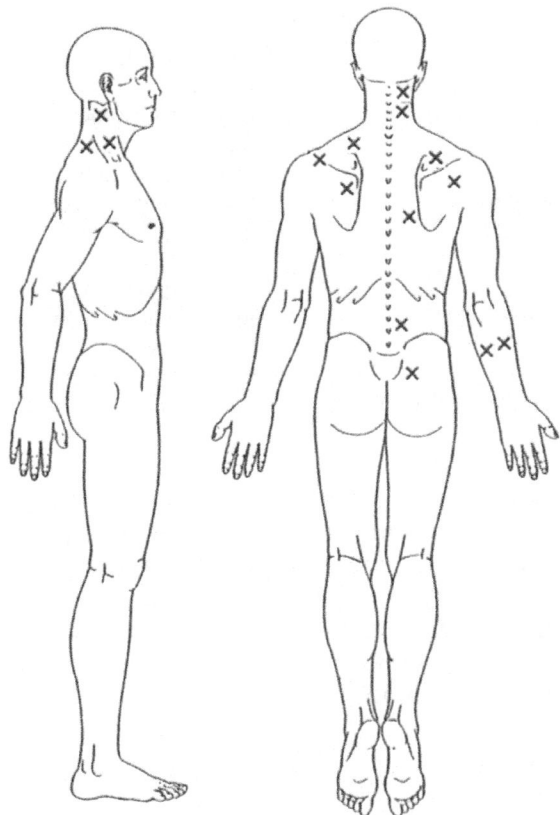

FIGURE 2.1. Common myofascial trigger points. The region of muscle that exhibits such marked tenderness is remarkably small. The points are not fixed; the x's simply indicate where to start looking. Trigger points are less common in the lower extremity. (From Travell, J. G., & Simons, D. G. 1983. Myofascial Pain and Dysfunction: The Trigger Point Manual. Copyright 1983 by Williams & Wilkins. Original figure reprinted with permission.)

TABLE 2.1. Common patterns of referred pain.

Vertex Pain	Frontal Headache
Sternocleidomastoid	frontalis
Splenius capitis	GON[a] entrapment
Occipital Pain	Eye and Forehead
Trapezius	Sternocleidomastoid
Semispinalis	GON or occipitalis
Temporalis	Trapezius
Posterior Neck	Shoulder and Arm
Multifidi	supraspinatus (lateral shoulder)
Infraspinatus	infraspinatus (front shoulder)
Trapezius	Trapezius

[a]GON, greater occipital nerve.

can be described as myofascial pain. Table 2.1 gives some common patterns of referred pain from specific muscles. Interestingly, patients are almost never aware of their trigger points. The pain provoked by lying on an infraspinatus trigger point at night is perceived in the shoulder; a trapezius trigger point as occipital headache; and a gastrocnemius trigger point as pain in the foot.

Active Versus Latent Trigger Points

Trigger points are quite common and can be found in normal individuals who do not complain of pain. Although few controlled studies have been published on this condition, 50% of an Air Force recruit population had palpable trigger points. In 200 unselected asymptomatic adults, latent trigger points were found in more than 50% of shoulders, with 5% showing referred pain (Travell & Simons, 1983). Among responsible factors, Travell and Simons suggested that chronic dystonia (increased resting tone) in the muscle may result from overuse, postural imbalance, and psychic distress. Anecdotally, this seems true, for latent trigger points can be routinely found in Type A executives, "yuppie" investment bankers, and other hard drivers.

That trigger points can be found in many normal individuals, particularly those who work under a lot of stress, leads to the distinction between active versus latent trigger points. Although much was made of this in earlier literature, it merely serves to distinguish between patients who spontaneously report pain and those who are surprised at the discomfort felt when the physician palpates a taut trigger point. I do not advise injecting latent trigger points, but only those found in patients who spontaneously complain of pain.

Clinical Diagnosis and Physical Examination

The diagnostic criteria for myofascial trigger points are found in Table 2.2. As an example, a history of chronic daily headache, neck pain, or back pain, with or without referred pain in the extremity, should prompt the physician to examine for myofascial trigger points. The method is quite simple. The examination begins with observation of posture, movement, and body structure and symmetry, and proceeds with palpation for active trigger points. With the patient seated, the physician palpates the common locations in the head, neck, and shoulders—these include the suboccipital, posterior, and lateral triangles of the neck; the midtrapezius at its superior border, and the infrascapular region. In the lower back, this includes the paraspinous musculature over the transverse processes and the multifidus triangle. These

TABLE 2.2. Diagnostic criteria for myofascial trigger points.

1. Exquisite *point* tenderness.
2. Reproduction of the parent's pain on palpation; often with a distinct pattern of referred pain.
3. Jump sign: Recoil, pain, and vocalization disproportionate to the pressure exerted on the trigger point.
4. Presence of a taut, palpable band.
5. Limitation of movement.

are the most common sites, and the primary physician will see them repeatedly.

Common mechanical stresses that precipitate trigger points include wrenching or twisting movements, auto accidents, falls, and sprains. In addition to grossly traumatic events involving a sudden overload or sustained muscular contraction, poor body mechanics while lifting or prolonged immobility, such as sitting belted in a plane or car, may activate paraspinous trigger points. Specifically, sustained spine flexion while working at a low desk can overload the posterior cervical muscles; too low or no armrests can overload the upper trapezius; the supraspinatus can be activated by carrying heavy packages, or being walked by the dog. Athletic persons may activate trigger points by lifting above shoulder height with the arm extended (e.g., military presses).

Most Common Symptomatic Complaints

The general principles of diagnosis and examination can be conveyed by looking at the most common symptomatic complaints, namely, headache, neck, and back pain.

Headache is referred pain produced by chronic myodystonia. The diagnostic term dystonia is used to refer to a sustained contraction of skeletal muscles that increases the resting tone, can be felt on physical examination and causes a characteristic aching pain. In lay terms, this is called muscle spasm. The headache is occipital or posterior neck or both, and with time may become generalized. The pain is a dull, monotonous ache that worsens as the day wears on and tends to be symmetrical. Because the greater and lesser occipital nerves pierce the nuchal musculature, the increase in muscle tone may, if chronic and severe enough, produce a secondary occipital neuralgia. The mechanism is similar to compression neuropathy. With this development, the pain radiates to the forehead, either above or behind the eye. Many patients explain their pain as eyestrain or other ocular problems and may seek to remedy it with new spectacles.

TABLE 2.3. Nerve entrapments from myofascial bands.[a]

Nerve	Muscle
Greater occipital	Semispinalis capitis
Supraorbital	Frontalis
Sensory radial	Brachialis
Deep radial	Supinator
Ulnar	Flexor carpi ulnaris
Brachial plexus	Scaleni, pectoralis minor
Posterior rami	Paraspinal muscles

[a]From Travell, J.G., Simons, D.G. 1983. Myofascial Pain and Dysfunction: The Trigger Point Manual. Copyright 1983 by Williams & Wilkins. Reprinted with permission.

There is nothing wrong with their eyes, however; the patients are merely misinterpreting the referred pain. Table 2.3 lists nerves commonly entrapped as they pass through taut bands of muscle fibers or between a band and bone.

Examination of persons with such a headache reveals trigger points in the suboccipital and posterior triangles of the neck. There may also be trigger points over the transverse processes of one or more cervical vertebrae and in the middle of the superior border of the trapezius. Firm pressure on these points, which are felt as a hard nodule or a palpable band in the muscle, causes two things: First, it reproduces the patient's headache or neck pain and, second, causes them to jump (jump sign). Such involuntary reaction, often with vocalization, is another reason why these painful spots are called trigger points.

When the occipital nerve has become irritated it will be very sensitive to palpation. The greater occipital nerve lies next to the occipital artery, whose pulse can be felt over the nuchal ridge midway between the inion (occipital protuberance) and the mastoid process (see Figure 4.1). Mild pressure on the nerve will reproduce the patient's headache, including its radiation to the forehead or eye. Patients should be asked directly, "Is this what your headache feels like?"

so that you can be certain about the diagnosis. Normal subjects can withstand considerable pressure on the nerve without discomfort. The technique of occipital nerve block is discussed in Chapter 4.

Additional trigger points in the upper back include the midrhomboid, scapular fossa, interscapular region, and Erb's point. Interesting enough, palpation here may cause referred pain in an extremity, even as far as the fingers, and myofascial pain may thereby be confused with a herniated disk. Although this is well known to clinicians, a mechanism for this referred pain is lacking. Injection of the trigger point will resolve the sensory dysesthesias in the arm. It is far easier to try this approach before working up a patient for cervical disk.

In the lumbar spine the most common points are over the transverse processes of the L4 to S1 vertebrae and the multifidus triangle. Palpation of these firm nodules reproduces the patient's pain. Referred pain is much more common in the upper extremities than into the legs.

Treatment

Treatment involves injection of a few milliliters of 0.25% bupivacaine into the point. Often, injection of one point will reflexly cause resolution of several of them. For example, if a patient with posterior headaches has trigger points in the suboccipital triangle, over the transverse process of C4, and in the midtrapezii bilaterally, injection of the midtrapezius points may release the dystonia in the other regions. In other words, it is not necessary to inject every point found on the physical exam. Because the points are often bilateral, both trapezii can be injected with a total of 10 ml of 0.25% bupivacaine with excellent results.

In the lower back, the physician can palpate along the paraspinous musculature of the lower lumbar vertebrae, calling out a number to the patient with each spot that he palpates.

The patient is instructed to decide which of the numbered spots is most painful. The most painful spot is the one injected; 5 to 10 ml of 0.25% bupivacaine with a 1.5-in. needle is recommended.

The general technique involves a sterile technique and injecting 1 to 5 ml of 0.25% bupivacaine until the point tenderness disappears and the patient's pain resolves. There is no need to use epinephrine. In the neck and upper back, a 1- to 1.5-in., 23-gauge needle is recommended; in the back or gluteal region, a 1.5- to 2-in., 21-gauge needle is used.

Because patients often have a fear of "needles," recumbency helps to both relax the muscle and prevent psychogenic syncope. The patient is told that if he can stand you pushing on the trigger point, then the injection feels no worse. This is generally true, although when the needle impales the trigger point there is sometimes a flash of pain.

In palpating trigger points, one sometimes wonders exactly what muscle is giving rise to the pain and how deep one should inject. At the level of C5, for example, a 2-in. needle will not penetrate the full depth of the posterior cervical muscles as long as it does not indent the skin. The rule of thumb is that enough anesthetic should be injected to remove the pain. If 2 to 3 ml superficially does not resolve the trigger point, then the needle should be advanced and aspirated, and injection continued until 5 to 8 ml have been injected in any one site. The syringe should always be aspirated before injecting to ensure the needle has not entered a vessel. Injection should never be done if blood enters the syringe at aspiration; arterial injection of only 2 ml of anesthetic has caused convulsions.

Pain relief occurs within seconds. Patients are often amazed that their chronic pain disappears so fast. After the injection, the muscle should be passively or actively stretched. If the problem is particularly severe or chronic, then hot packs can be applied. I prefer to use them for 15 minutes before injecting, as their use after injection seems, through increased blood flow, to dissipate the anesthetic quickly. A firm, kneading manual massage is also a helpful ancillary procedure.

Travell recommends recording trigger points and any pattern of referred pain on an anatomical chart such as the one in Figure 2.1. This is particularly useful in the patient complaining of "no improvement." A new drawing is compared with the first one to see whether there is in fact a change in the location of trigger points and pain. If pain relief was complete for some hours or days, despite its return, you can then assure the patient that a muscular cause has been established and that it can be ultimately relieved. Patients need tangible evidence that the pain originates in the muscles rather than in arthritis, in pinched nerves, or in their mind. With injection, exercise, good posture, and modest physical therapy, they can resolve their problem. If the principle were not routinely violated it would not need saying that bupivacaine injections address the cause of pain whereas analgesic pills merely mask the pain. If medication were to be prescribed, the a muscle relaxer such as chlorzoxazone (Parafon Forte) would be a logical choice.

Terms such as tendonitis, tennis elbow, and anterior compartment syndrome have been used to describe trigger-point pain in the extremities. The generalist is likely to see these complaints often. The principle for trigger point injection is the same as for the neck and back, although the dose is less: 1 to 3 ml of 0.25% bupivacaine will suffice.

Trigger Points After Injury

One routinely finds trigger points in patients who have sustained injuries such as sporting accidents, work mishaps, or automobile accidents. It is perhaps easier to understand them in the context of injury than the spontaneous variety that arise in the course of normal activity. Symptoms often are not immediate; persistent pain and stiffness appear after a day's delay.

Being a neurologist, I see a good deal of trauma. It is surprising how often the family physician or even specialists fail to examine the patient for focal myodystonia. It is almost a regular occurrence. I hope that this handbook will lead primary practitioners to examine for this condition in this setting, thus preventing patients from going many months with chronic pain. In the classic automobile accident, the laws of physics dictate that the head moves toward the impact. Thus, with a stationary driver who is rear ended, there will first be a hyperextension of the neck and then a brisk flexion. This sudden and violent muscular and ligamentous stretch sets up the mechanical events for dystonia. After the flexion there is usually a rebound extension, with the occipital nerves often sustaining blunt trauma on the headrest. Because of the design of shoulder belts, the trunk torts to the left, and the left occipital nerve is injured more often than the right on the rebound. The diagnosis of occipital neuralgia is mentioned previously, and the technique of occipital nerve block is discussed in Chapter 4.

With a moving driver who sustains a front-end collision, the sequence of events is the opposite: a forward flexion and then rapid hyperextension, often with blunt trauma to the occipital nerves and suboccipital muscles against the headrest. It is worth mentioning that in classic "whiplash" the anterior neck is always injured. Malingerers point to the back of their neck where they think their neck bones are, whereas patients examined in the *acute* phase will always have anterior cervical problems and may acknowledge dysphagia or change in voice when directly asked. The sternal insertion of the sternocleidomastoid or the collis muscle may be strained or torn. There may be loss of the laryngeal "click" as it slides over the vertebral body secondary to edema or retropharyngeal hematoma.

Unfortunately, the biomechanical factors that cause injury in impact trauma are known to the majority of automotive engineers but only a fraction of physicians. For example, whiplash was recognized in World War II when pilots of catapult take-off craft had to discharged from service because of intractable neck pain, vertigo, and occasional symptoms of concussion. The solution was to extend the seat back to support the head. Automotive designers later became aware of this and introduced headrests to prevent hyperextension of the neck. Nonetheless, injury to the neck is quite common in this setting and results from tensile, shear, and compressive strains resulting from a combination of overbending, axial compression, and rotational loads. There is also, as was mentioned, frequent rebound impact with injury to the occipital nerves and suboccipital muscles. The reader interested in this topic should consult Cytowic, Stump & Larned (1988) and Viano (1988).

Further Reading

Travell, J., Simons D. G. 1983. Myofascial Pain and Dysfunction: The Trigger Point Manual. Baltimore: Williams & Wilkins.
(Details of muscular anatomy can be found in standard anatomy texts.)

3 —

General Techniques and Indications

General Indications

There are certain general principles that should be followed in evaluating all patients with pain. It is obvious that lack of attention to general principles is the cause of misdiagnosis and mismanagement of specific pain syndromes yet such general principles are routinely violated.

The medical and neurological examination should lead to a correct diagnosis. Specific maneuvers or procedures can then confirm that diagnosis. Should the patient be in severe pain at the time of the initial evaluation, adequate analgesics will easily permit him to participate in the evaluation. Pain should never be an excuse not to thoroughly examine a patient. Reassessment is necessary if the response is less than expected, or if pain returns to its original level. A series of a few blocks may provide long-term relief.

Generally, nerve block should be considered when (a) oral medications are obviously not helping or when large, continuous doses of narcotics are needed to suppress pain; (b) the pain has a focal anatomical localization; and (c) the pain is chronic and severe. Beyond treatment, local nerve blocks are also useful for diagnosis and prognosis.

In the previous chapter (Chapter 2), we discussed the indications for and technique of myofascial pain. In this chapter we talk about general considerations of true nerve block. Those that the primary physician will find useful and be able to perform himself involve blockade of superficial nerves of the head and scalp, spinal and intercostal nerves (e.g., postherpetic neuralgia), cervical and lumbar radiculopathies, peripheral neuropathies (e.g., diabetic), and entrapment neuropathies (carpal tunnel). Sympathetic blocks interrupt the vicious cycle of hyperpathia and chronic pain seen in reflex sympathetic dystrophy and sympathetically mediated pain.

A big reason why nerve block is not more popular and why pain patients suffer needlessly is that their diagnostic work-up is commonly quite poor. Diagnosis and treatment should always be paired. In the bulk of cases the outcome should be successful if the diagnosis is correct. The diagnosis (*dia* = through, *gnosis* = knowledge) of pain relies most on the history, somewhat on the physical examination, and little if at all on machine tests. Unfortunately, chronic pain patients become labeled "intractable" when they fail to respond to the same old treatments (read pills), as if the same action should somehow produce different results. Having failed to remedy the problem, the physician then invites the patient to seek psychiatric care. As I suggested in Chapter 1, a positive rather than negative physician attitude greatly enhances the results of nerve block.

Patients have a different concept of analgesia than doctors and nurses do. They expect a relatively constant level of relief. The patient who experiences several hour-long peaks of pain will judge the treatment not helpful.

Other Indications

Although not discussed in this handbook, some nerve block procedures should be kept in mind. The orthopedist should consider nerve blocks with various fractures, such as femoral nerve block for fractured femur, and brachial plexus block for fractured humerous. Even a single rib fracture can be very painful, and relief can be obtained by intercostal nerve block.

The internist should consider anesthesia consultation for epidural block or lumbar sympathectomy for urinary calculi, and celiac plexus or splanchnic block for acute pancreatitis and other abdominal pains.

Positive and Negative Effects of Nerve Blocks

The beneficial effects of nerve block were mentioned under the general principles presented in Table 1.1. These involve interruption of the pain at or near its source, interruption of abnormal reflexes, blockade of sympathetic hyperactivity and improvement of blood flow, enhancement of the doctor–patient relationship in the context of the overall treatment strategy, and gaining patient cooperation in exploring psychological issues by the attention to the physical aspect of the patient's pain.

On the negative side, presenting nerve block as simply a technical intervention may reinforce some patients' conviction (usually those patients with high behavior and low medical findings) that they are sick, fostering both dependence and passivity. Such patients may be at higher risk for nocebo responses (discussed later in this chapter). Finally, nerve blocks are an invasive procedure and do carry the risk of some moderate complications when improperly performed.

Choice and Concentration of Anesthetic Agent

I mentioned in Chapter 1 that both saline injection and dry-needling (acupuncture) do produce anesthesia, although their effectiveness pales when compared to a true anesthetic. Although Travell historically used procaine, arguing that it had fewer systemic and myotoxic effects in addition to its curare-like effect on the myoneural junction, experience has shown that the long-acting aminoacyl anesthetics, such as bupivicaine and etidocaine, provide superior and longer lasting pain relief. These anesthetics contain an amide linkage between the aromatic nucleus and the piperidine group; procaine-type anesthetics have an ester linkage. Procaine has the briefest duration of action and is associated with allergic reactions.

Bupivacaine blocks the generation and conduction of nerve impulses by slowing propagation and reducing the rate of rise of the action potential. It also increases the threshold for electrical stimulation. Anesthesia is related to the diameter, myelination, and conduction velocity of the nerve fibers. Clinically, a progressive loss of function occurs in the following order: pain, temperature, touch, proprioception, then skeletal muscle tone.

The duration of nerve block is proportional to the dose of bupivacaine. Thus, higher concentrations of bupivacaine

TABLE 3.1. Average dose and volume of bupivacaine.[a]

Type of block	Concentration (%)	Average (ml)	Average (mg)
Trigger-point–field anesthesia	0.25	3–20	7.5–50, to 150 maximum
Large muscles (e.g., lumbar, trapezius)	0.5	5–10	25–50, to 150 maximum
Peripheral nerve	0.25	3–10	7.5–25
Stellate ganglion sympathetic	0.25	20	50

[a]The author's maximum recommended dose for the types of blocks discussed in the handbook is 150 mg. The manufacturer's maximum human daily dose for Marcaine brand of bupivacaine is 400 mg.

will provide longer relief. The possibility of systemic side effects, however, should be kept in mind. I recommend only 0.25% and 0.5% bupivacaine because complete sensory block is achieved with the lesser concentrations for 18 to 24 hours. Pain relief lasts far longer than the pharmacologic sensory block.

Because the effect on motor function depends on concentration, the 0.25% solution will not produce complete motor block. The production of motor block is not particularly germane to the treatment of the pain syndromes, however. Therefore, for most purposes, 0.25% bupivacaine will be sufficient. In large persons or when injecting large muscles, the 0.5% solution may be used to reduce the necessary volume. In the paralumbar muscles, for example, 5 ml of 0.5% bupivacaine can be used at each injection site (see Table 3.1).

It is my impression that many specialists, particularly orthopedists, like to add a steroid to the anesthetic. I cannot find good controlled studies showing that this combination is actually superior to bupivacaine alone. We must consider such evidence anecdotal. The theoretical reason for using steroids is that it is a strong antiinflammatory agent. It logically follows that steroids may be helpful in conditions that truly involve inflammation. In my own experience, I use steroids only in median nerve block for carpal tunnel, because oral antiinflammatories (prednisone, NSAIDs) benefit perhaps 20% of patients. Two steroids commonly used are dexamethasone, at 4 mg per 10 ml of anesthetic, and triamcinolone (Kenalog) 0.2%.

Preparing the Patient

It is beneficial for the primary physician to perform nerve block and trigger-point injection because he or she is more than a technical specialist who just inserts needles. A therapeutic relationship will be already established, and the practitioner will have had ample time for examination and diagnosis. The neurological elements of that examination are also the baseline against which the effects of the block will be compared.

The patient should understand the reason for the procedure and what you hope will be accomplished by it. This is an elective procedure and should never be forced on the patient. The patient should have time to think about the block and consider any alternatives. Most patients readily agree to do it on the spot when the physician presents nerve block as the option he recommends. The patient is told that the block will be followed by a short course of medication or physical therapy. Severity of pain is a particularly good reason to recommend nerve block. If the patient rates the pain "10" on a scale of 10, then pills are likely to have little effect. After the block completely knocks out the pain, it usually returns at a much lesser level, and pills can then be much more effective. Sometimes the pain may not return at all, but if it does then a few further blocks may resolve the problem.

Nonetheless, initial resistance is seen often enough that the physician should have a well-thought-out plan to counter it. Resistance from "fear of needles" should be countered by information and reassurance, not brute force or appeal to authority. Patients should understand, however, that the longer the pain is untreated the more difficult it will be to treat *by any method*. This is particularly important for patients who ask to try supposedly more benign alternatives such as pills.

For example, a patient with severe daily posterior headaches, with bifrontal or retroorbital radiation, may certainly be allowed to try alternatives such as muscle relaxers, antiinflammatories, or carbamezapine (Tegretol). The effect of such alternatives is likely to be nil, however, if the occipital nerves are tender to palpation. Further, simply masking the pain with narcotic analgesics does little to treat its cause. Such fearful patients are best served by probing and countering their fears; for example, you are not going to stick a needle into their head (a rather common assumption!) but under the skin, and the injection itself feels no worse than the pain evoked by pressing on the nerve, which by now you have already done several times.

The difference in rationale between therapeutic and prognostic blocks should be carefully explained. If, for example, a median nerve block for carpal tunnel is proposed to see whether surgery is indicated, patients may be disappointed that the relief is only temporary if they have not understood this before the procedure. It should also be emphasized that sometimes several blocks are necessary before a notable dent is made in their pain. The patient will need to evaluate not only the immediate effects but also those over the course of several days or weeks.

Placebo and Nocebo Responses

In Chapter 2 I mentioned that both bupivacaine nerve block and saline injection (an impure placebo) involved the endogenous opioid system and could be reversed by naloxone. Because there is a demonstrable placebo response in addition to the pharmacologic action of bupivacaine, the physician may wish to take advantage of it. Unfortunately, some physicians are somewhat hostile to placebo interventions, equating them with deception. When viewed as a symbolic input to the healing intervention, however, the deliberate evocation of an ancillary placebo response can be viewed as quite ethical in the doctor–patient relationship, particularly when it permits weaning the patient away from physical dependence on drugs.

We read in Chapter 1 that injections are superior to pills, and a better response is obtained when the physician has a positive, optimistic attitude, and suggests that a strong analgesic is being given that will definitely relieve the pain for a long time.

A nocebo response is an untoward event that cannot be explained by physiology or pharmacology. The complaint is usually bizarre, nonanatomical, and may escalate with time. Such bizarre impairments may last for days after nerve block. Examples are bilateral numbness when only one side has been injected; paralysis, extremely unlikely with less than 0.75% bupivacaine in doses under 100 mg; and subjective swelling. Nocebo phenomena are likely to be seen in patients who have high pain behavior and low medical findings (Brena, 1985).

Follow-Up Treatment After Block

Some type of short-term or as-needed treatment is usually prescribed after nerve block. If the pain is myofascial, this could include muscle relaxers (particularly chlorzoxazone/APAP) and physical therapy. Effective therapy involves heat, manual massage, and stretching exercises, in that order. For neuritic pain, conventional treatments involve tricyclic agents or anticonvulsants that suppress peripheral nerve conduction. Among the tricyclics I prefer imipramine (Tofranil) at 50 to 150 mg h.s. While much has been written about the usefulness of amitriptyline (Elavil) in doses much less then those used for depression (i.e., 10–50 mg h.s.), I find so many people complain of sedation that I personally do not use it. Dilantin at 200 to 300 mg daily is inexpensive and will have an effect within 5 days if it helps at all; carbamezapine (Tegretol), however, is usually more effective at 100 to 300 b.i.d. Some patients are reassured by having an analgesic they can fall back on in case nothing else works.

Adverse Effects and Contraindications

Despite their good safety record and the experience gained by familiarity, local anesthetics are not entirely benign. "Local" anesthetics are systemically absorbed, and the practitioner must be familiar with anticipated adverse effects, complications, and contraindications. To be sure, adverse effects are much more common with epidural and spinal anesthesia, obstetric uses, and procedures involving the head (e.g., retrobulbar block, dental anesthesia); these topics are not considered in this handbook. Instead, I focus on peripheral nerve and myofascial trigger-point injections, the safest and most common of the various anesthetic nerve block procedures.

Systemic absorption of bupivacaine affects mainly the cardiovascular and central nervous systems. At serum concentrations achieved with customary doses, these effects are minimal if ever seen. Toxic concentrations, however, can depress cardiac conduction and excitability, leading to atrioventricular (AV) block, ventricular arrythmias, and cardiac arrest. There is further peripheral vasodilitation leading to hypotension and decreased cardiac output. Such cardiovascular changes are most likely to occur with unintentional intravascular injection. For this reason, both incremental dosage and frequent aspiration are advised.

Bupivacaine, like all local anesthetics, primarily depresses the central nervous system (CNS) at toxic doses. Respiratory arrest may result from medullary suppression. Depression is sometimes preceded by an excited state of restlessness, tremors, and convulsion. Again, this is seen primarily with intravascular, especially intraarterial, injection.

The rate of systemic absorption is proportional to the total dose (therefore, concentration) as well as the vascularity of the injection site. Although bupivacaine with epinephrine reduces the rate of absorption and peak plasma concentration, I do not recommend bupivacaine with epinephrine except for intercostal block. The use of epinephrine, a vasoconstrictor, may lead to ischemia or tissue necrosis in tissues served by end arteries (nose, ear, penis, digits).

Following peripheral nerve block injection into muscle, peak levels of bupivacaine occur in 30 to 45 minutes and wane over 3 to 6 hours. The half-life of bupivacaine is 2.7 hours. A rapid injection of a large volume should be avoided. Incremental doses should be used when possible. Multidose vials that contain antimicrobial agents should not be used for stellate ganglion block.

The absolute contraindication to the use of bupivacaine is a known hypersensitivity to it or other amide local anesthetics. Bupivacaine is contraindicated in obstetrical paracervical block, as such use has caused fetal bradycardia or death. Allergic reactions are quite rare and result from sensitivity to bupivicaine or the preservative (methylparaben) included in multidose vials. Allergic reactions consist of such common phenomena as urticaria, angioneurotic edema (including laryngeal edema), bronchial constriction, tachycardia, hypotension, nausea, and dizziness. Hypersensitivity to local anesthetics, itself quite rare, seems to occur most often with ester-type compounds (e.g., procaine and tetracaine).

Due attention should be paid to avoiding complications in the first place. This involves maintaining a sterile technique, incremental dose injection, aspiration before injection (particularly when the needle has been advanced), and monitoring the patient for those adverse effects which are most common.

General procedures such as recumbency and evaluation of the legs should be first used in hypotension. Pressor drugs and fluids should be immediately available. Angioneurotic edema may require the use of epinephrine or atropine. If an adequate airway is not achieved by extending the neck and elevating the jaw, than an oral airway, face mask, or intubation may be necessary depending on the clinical situation. Other measures should be undertaken by those familiar with their use and should be immediately available.

It should be again emphasized that untoward cardiac and CNS effects are almost always seen with intravascular or subarachnoid injection. In these instances, shock, cardiac and respiratory arrest, and convulsions may be seen. Should this inadvertent reaction occur, assuring an adequate airway is of primary importance. Oxygen administration lessens the likelihood of convulsions. Patients who do show anesthetic-induced convulsions rapidly develop hypoxia, hypercarbia, and acidosis within minutes of onset. The immediate treatment of these systemic derangements may lessen the likelihood of cardiac arrest. Mean plasma dosage of bupivacaine needed to induce seizures in rhesus monkeys is 4.4 mg/kg.

Use During Pregnancy

Bupivacaine is widely used at term for obstetrical anesthesia. However, there are not adequate data on the possible effect of bupivacaine on the developing fetus. Embryocidal effects in animals are seen with five times with maximum daily human dose of 400 mg. Bupivacaine crosses the placenta by passive diffusion, which is governed by the degree of plasma protein binding, drug ionization, and lipid solubility. With a protein-binding capacity of 95%, bupivacaine therefore has a low ratio of fetal/maternal concentration. In the absence of well-controlled studies in pregnant women, the practitioner will have to weigh the potential benefit against the risk.

I have used bupivacaine blocks at minimal effective doses after the first trimester, primarily in trigger-point, occipital nerve, and paraspinal block in lieu of opting for regular doses of analgesics or other drugs. In this setting, occasional nerve block with a physical therapy program has been effective treatment.

It is not known whether local anesthetics, including bupivacaine, are excreted in human milk, although many drugs are. Again, benefits must be weighed against the risks. The manufacturer does not recommend bupivacaine in children under 12 years.

Additional information about the Marcaine brand of bupi-vacaine is found in the package insert, with which the physician should be thoroughly familiar.

4 —
Specific Applications

Blocks for Headache

Headache is among the top five conditions for which people seek medical attention. The principle I would like to emphasize is that of rational treatment. That is, it makes far more sense to apply a specific treatment to a specific type of headache (diagnostic entity) than to throw a favorite nostrum indiscriminately at all headaches. I assume the practitioner can distinguish migraine and its variants and treat it with specific antimigraine drugs such as ergots or beta blockers. To prescribe narcotics as a first choice is not only irrational but poor practice.

Likewise, there are specific headaches that respond beautifully to bupivacaine injection, and treating them so is most appropriate because it addresses the cause of the headache rather than merely masking the pain.

The compact anatomy of the head and neck demands accurate placement of the needle and small doses of anesthetic for effective and safe pain relief. Fortunately, landmarks are easily found. The practitioner may wish to consult standard anatomy texts in addition to the diagrams in this book for further detail. Incorrect placement of the needle is usually the reason for failure. Review of the anatomy just before the procedure may be advisable.

The diagnostic considerations and techniques for specific applications follow.

Greater Occipital Nerve Block

Occipital neuralgia is rather common, although few physicians are aware of it; and if my personal education is typical, students and residents are not taught how to examine for it. The two most common circumstances in which you will see it are in patients with frequent tension headaches (chronic daily headache), and in injury cases (auto accidents, falls, work mishaps).

The pain is a monotonous ache in the back of the head with spikes of paroxysmal pain that are referred to the forehead or eye. With a focal injury the headache is unilateral; with whiplash and chronic daily headache, it becomes bilateral with time. When due to blunt trauma, the headache is usually worse in the morning if the patient customarily sleeps on his back. If the result of entrapment by cervical myodystonia, the headache tends to intensify as the day wears on and the associated dystonia worsens.

Begin the examination by palpating the midline of the superior border of the trapezius; then the posterior, lateral, and suboccipital triangles in the neck; and last, the occipital nerve, observing for the jump sign (usually rather marked when present) and the patient's acknowledgment of pain during these maneuvers. The greater occipital nerve (GON) lies midway between the mastoid process and inion (occipital protuberance at the midline), adjacent to the occipital artery whose pulse can be palpated after some practice. The lesser occipital nerve is 1 to 2 cm lateral to this (Figure 4.1).

Because occipital neuralgia and cervical myodystonia often coexist, it is important to distinguish which is more important in the individual patient and which condition, therefore, you will treat. Digital pressure on the nerve can easily generate 5 pounds per square inch, which bothers no one. Perhaps one-fifth this pressure is exquisitely painful to patients with occipital neuralgia. The important feature is that such manual pressure on the nerve exactly reproduces the quality and anterior radiation of their headache. Patients should be directly asked, "Is this what your headache feels like?" If the palpation of trigger points in the neck and shoulder girdle is more uncomfortable, then any occipital neuralgia is likely secondary and the patient will benefit more from trigger-point injection and treatment of the dystonia.

An alternative method for locating the nerve if the artery cannot be felt is blind palpation. The nerve underlies the site where palpation reproduces the patient's pain.

For blockade of the GON alone, either unilateral or bilateral, a 5-ml syringe is filled with 0.25% bupivicaine and fitted with a $\frac{5}{8}$-in. 25-gauge needle. The patient is prone with a

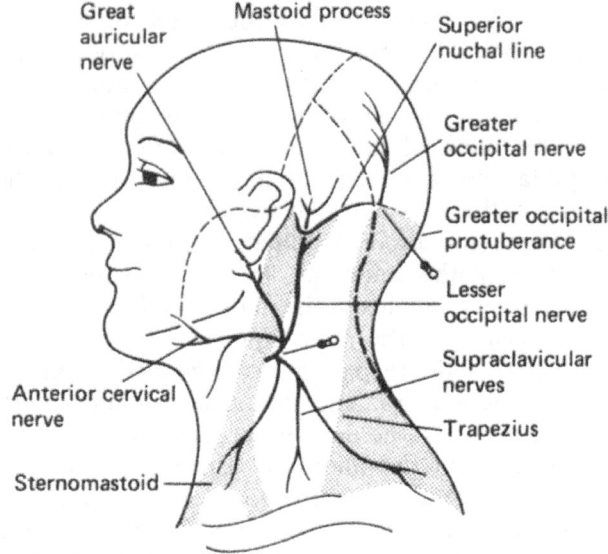

FIGURE 4.1. The superficial cervical plexus emerges at the midpoint of the posterior border of the sternocleidomastoid, superficial to the deep fascia. Superficial infiltration here produces anesthesia of the side of the head and neck. See text for further details. From Murphy, T. 1980. Neural Blockade, 1st edition, Cousins & Bridenbaugh (eds.), p. 421. Copyright 1980 by Lippincott. Reprinted with permission.

small pillow or roll half under the chest and half under the chin to take tension off the posterior cervical muscles. The physician stands on the patient's left side. The first and third fingers of the left hand rest on the mastoid and inion, respectively, and the index finger bisects this distance to approximate the location of the GON and occipital artery. The right index finger then palpates for the artery and once found, firm pressure over this area again confirms reproduction of the patient's headache. The left index finger can then mark this position while the right is free to prep the area and perform the actual injection.

Needle entry is just lateral to the pulse with the tip pointing superiorly or somewhat laterally depending on preference. Aspirate before injecting 1 to 3 ml of bupivacaine in incremental doses. Incremental dosing is desirable for two reasons. First, the dystonic muscles are themselves painful and sensitive to the sting of the advancing edge of anesthetic. Second, good block can be established with rather small doses of bupivacaine; rarely is the entire 5 ml necessary. After 30 to 60 seconds, with the needle still in place, the left hand tests sensation on the injected side from the occiput to the vertex with a sharp object (broken applicator stick or sterile 16-gauge needle) to determine the effectiveness of the block. A good block develops rapidly over 1 to 3 minutes. Sensation is compared to the uninjected side, and more bupivacaine is injected if required. With practice, a good block is produced with about 2.5 ml. Patients should be told not to worry about the lump that they will feel for a few days.

Blockade of both the greater and lesser occipital nerves on one side is accomplished with the same volume but using a 1.5-in., 23-gauge needle. Injection is about 2 cm lateral to the occipital artery with the syringe held parallel to the skin surface. Always aspirating before injecting; the 5 ml is deposited across the nuchal ridge.

Sensory blockade will last for 18 to 24 hours. Pain relief, on the other hand, lasts at least a day, often much longer, up to a week or sometimes permanently. If the pain does return, it usually does so at a much lower level. Should this occur and be severe enough to warrant further treatment, repeat blocks can be done every 1 to 3 weeks. If the problem is not resolved by 3 blocks and the occipital nerves remain tender, I recommend carbamezapine (Tegretol), 200 to 600 mg. total daily for 4 to 12 weeks.

Superficial Cervical Plexus Block

Unilateral temporal headaches or neck pain may be abolished by blocking the superficial cervical plexus. This involves a needle insertion at the midpoint of the posterior border of the sternocleidomastoid (SCM) muscle (see Figure 4.1). The superficial cervical plexus consists of the anterior rami of C2–C4 superficial to the deep fascia of the neck. At the point of emergence, the plexus divides into four nerves: the lesser occipital, greater auricular, anterior cervical cutaneous, and supraclavicular.

The posterior border of the SCM is easily palpated, and superficial infiltration of 3 to 10 ml of 0.25% bupivicaine is done. An important neighboring structure is the spinal accessory nerve, which emerges just above the superficial cervical plexus. The accessory nerve, however, lies *deep* to the deep fascia of the neck, which should not be pierced during the block of the superficial plexus. The spinal accessory nerve is intentionally blocked at times to produce paralysis of the trapezius during shoulder operations.

Successful block of the superficial cervical plexus produces analgesia in the C2–C4 dermatomes laterally and anteriorly. While the greater and lesser occipital nerves can be blocked bilaterally at one sitting, I do not recommend bilateral superficial plexus blocks.

Temporalis Injection for Temporal Headaches

I did not specifically mention the temporalis muscle in Chapter 2 on myofascial pain. In patients with tension headaches or bruxism (teeth grinding), the temporalis may be exquisitely tender. Local infiltration of a few milliliters of bupivacaine can be done with a $\frac{5}{8}$-in., 25-gauge needle. The superficial temporal artery is palpated and the injection done posterior to it.

Neck Pain and Cervical Myodystonia: Tension Headache

Patients with generalized headaches will often be found to have rather marked cervical dystonia. Such patients are often hard drivers who engage in polyphasic behavior and are "too busy" for activities that might relax them such as vacations, athletics, meditation, and therapeutic massage. Such patients fit the stereotype of tension headache.

The most common sites for myofascial trigger points involve the suboccipital triangle, paracervical musculature over the transverse processes of C4–C5, and the midpoint of the upper trapezius. The difference between myofascial pain in the suboccipital triangle and tenderness of the GON is clearly distinguished by the physical examination. Injection in the suboccipital triangle is just below the nuchal ridge.

One should be properly concerned about inadvertent injection into an artery or vein in this region. With myofascial injections in the neck, including the suboccipital triangle, I use a 1-in., 23-gauge needle. As mentioned in Chapter 2, a 2-in. (5-cm) needle inserted at the level of C5 will not reach to the depth of the vertebral artery as long as it does not indent the skin (Travell & Simons, 1983, p. 316). Most injections are done in the superficial muscle layer at a 0.5- to 1.0-in. depth.

Carpal Tunnel Syndrome

Carpal tunnel syndrome (CTS), sometimes called repetitive motion syndrome, involves an entrapment of the median nerve at the wrist by the flexor retinaculum. Surgery for this condition should come, in my opinion, as a last resort and be reserved for cases in which motor weakness and atrophy have developed. Good results are never obtained with surgery in patients who only have pain. If this is accepted, then nerve block has a primary role in conservative management.

CTS is the most common peripheral nerve lesion. It is therefore particularly surprising to realize that this condition was first recognized only in the 1940s and put on a firm physiological basis by nerve conduction velocity measurements in the 1950s. Patten (1977) notes that some physicians

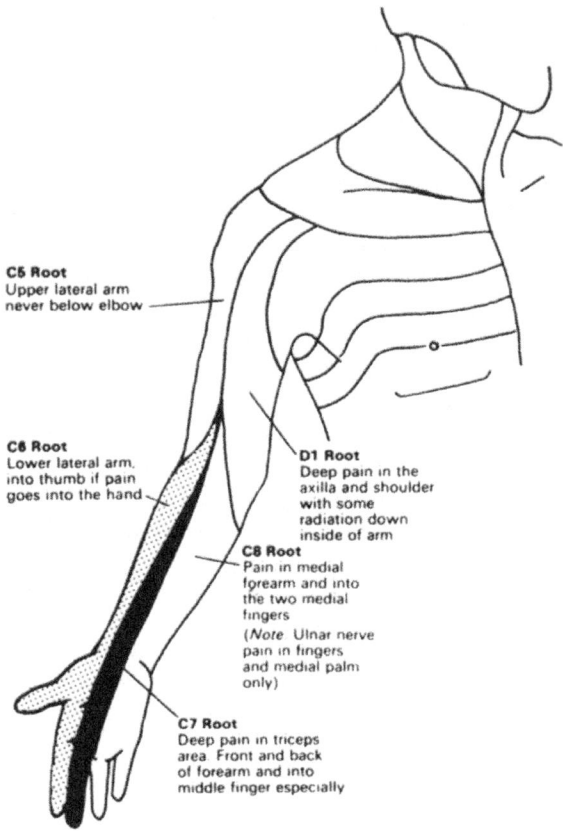

FIGURE 4.2. Characteristic pain patterns of peripheral nerves compared to those of root lesions. There is a wide disparity between what patients claim and what they ought to claim on purely anatomical grounds. From Patten, S. 1977. Neurological Differential Diagnosis, p. 177. Copyright 1977 by Springer-Verlag. Reprinted with permission.

"denied the existence of this condition for a whole decade after its original description and insisted that all pain in the hand was due to 'outlet syndromes'."

Figure 4.2 shows the distribution of pain in the hand. It is

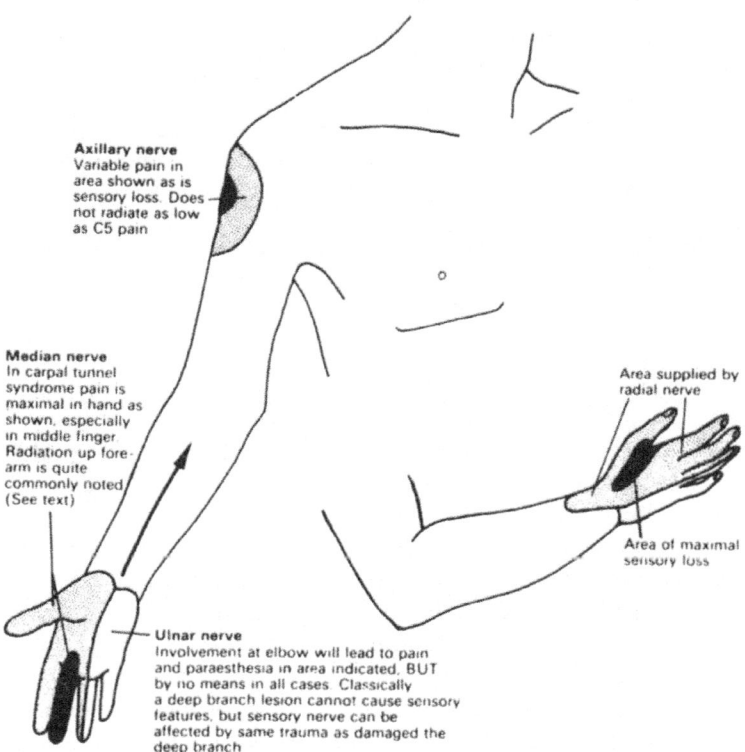

Axillary nerve
Variable pain in area shown as is sensory loss. Does not radiate as low as C5 pain

Median nerve
In carpal tunnel syndrome pain is maximal in hand as shown, especially in middle finger. Radiation up forearm is quite commonly noted (See text)

Area supplied by radial nerve

Area of maximal sensory loss

Ulnar nerve
Involvement at elbow will lead to pain and paraesthesia in area indicated, BUT by no means in all cases. Classically a deep branch lesion cannot cause sensory features, but sensory nerve can be affected by same trauma as damaged the deep branch

FIGURE 4.2 (*Continued*)

particularly severe at night, an important diagnostic feature. Conversely, cervical root pain is worse on awakening in the morning. Patten points out that on purely anatomical grounds compression of the median nerve at the wrist should cause pain only in the lateral palm and first three and a half fingers. Yet many patients insist that the pain shoots up into the forearm and elbow, sometimes even to the shoulder. Many also insist that *all* the fingers are involved, and this latter "nonanatomic" fact may have to do with the large number of sympathetic efferents to blood vessels in the

TABLE 4.1. Common causes of carpal tunnel syndrome (median nerve entrapment).

Repetitive Motion
    Repetitive flexion and extension of the wrist (assembly line workers, cafeteria workers, typists, musicians) or repetitive blows to the wrist (pneumatic drills, other machinery)
Trauma
    Sprains, fractures, and dislocations of carpal bones
Illness
    Myxedema, acromegaly, pregnancy, diabetes, amyloid, rheumatoid arthritis

hand, almost all of which travel in the median nerve. In addition to accounting for pain in all the fingers, it may also explain why some people insist that at the height of pain, the fingers blanch and swell. Such clinical facts are merely an instance of the common observation of the wide disparity between what *actually* happens and what *ought* to happen on purely anatomical grounds.

Many muscles supplied by the median nerve either have a dual innervation from the ulnar nerve or can be compensated for by the long forearm muscles. It is often only weakness and atrophy of the abductor pollicis brevis (thenar eminence) that can be demonstrated. Decreased touch and pin prick may be found over the radial palm and fingers, and the parasthetic pain may be reproduced by tapping over the nerve at the wrist (Tinel's sign). The diagnosis rests most heavily, however, on the characteristic pain and its distribution. Table 4.1 lists common causes of CTS.

Conventional treatment involves refraining from the repetitive activity that produced the entrapment in the first place, a cock-up splint (particularly at night), and anticonvulsants such as phenytoin and carbamezapine. The experienced clinician knows that these treatments do not help all cases; he also knows that the natural history favors spontaneous resolution of many cases. In those patients in whom there is no pain relief, and who are beginning to develop motor weak-

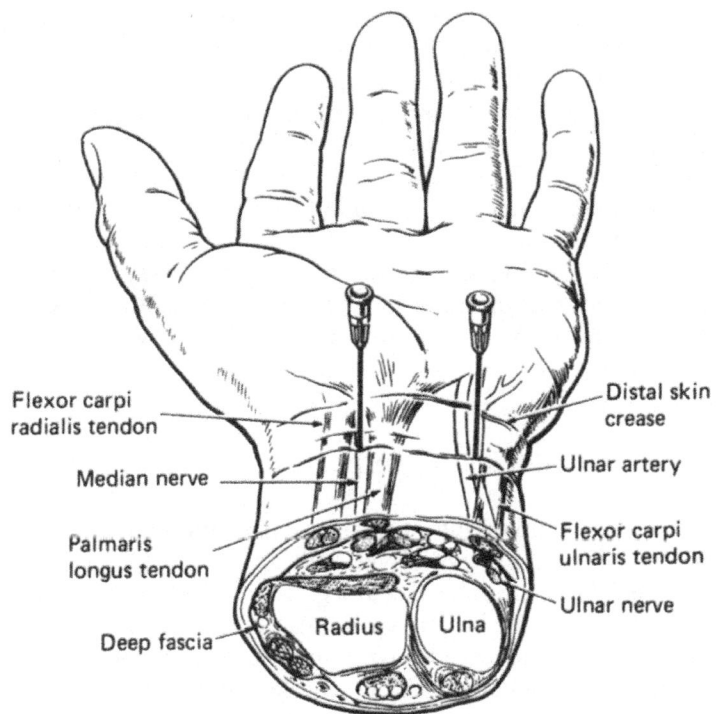

Flexor carpi
radialis tendon

Median nerve

Palmaris
longus tendon

Deep fascia

Distal skin
crease

Ulnar artery

Flexor carpi
ulnaris tendon

Ulnar nerve

Radius   Ulna

FIGURE 4.3. Anatomy for median nerve block. From Bridenbaugh, P. 1988. Neural Blockade, 1st edition, p. 409. Copyright 1988 by Lippincott. Reprinted with permission.

ness, median nerve block with bupivacaine and steroid often achieves gratifying results. In my own experience, nerve block often produces long-lasting results, stops progression to weakness, and may even be curative. Whether to truly attribute cure to the block itself, or any treatment for that matter, is difficult to know given the natural history. There are no well-controlled studies comparing block to surgery.

Technique: See Figure 4.3. The median nerve lies between the palmaris longus tendon and that of the flexor carpi radialis. These tendons are identified by flexing the wrist against resistance with the fingers extended. Needle insertion is done about 2 cm proximal to the proximal transverse wrist crease. With the wrist slightly extended, a $\frac{5}{8}$-in., 25-gauge needle is inserted perpendicularly to the skin between the tendons until it penetrates deep fascia; usually this is less than 1 cm deep.

Aspiration and incremental injection is performed. Intense parasthesias either on insertion or with injection of a very small volume suggests that the needle has impaled the nerve itself. The needle should be withdrawn slightly. Four milligrams of dexamethasone, 5 mg of triamcinolone (Kenalog), or 40 mg of methylprednisolone (Gilroy & Meyer, 1975) is added.

Intercostal Block for Herpes Zoster

Zoster is the unmasking of a latent virus that has been present ever since the original varicella infection. Chicken pox (varicella) and shingles (zoster) are caused by the same DNA virus. Zoster begins with pain, parasthesias, and dysesthesias in the affected dermatome, followed by vesicular eruptions in a few days. The vesicles scab over in 1 week and heal in a month's time. The dorsal root ganglion, dorsal horn of the cord, and meninges are the site of severe inflammation, hemorrhage, and necrosis. The peripheral nerve of the ganglion undergoes demylination, fibrosis, and cellular infiltration. Usually only a few segmental nerves are involved because immunity is renewed as the virus multiplies. The exception, of course, is in immunocompromised patients in whom multidermatomal zoster is seen.

There is a predilection for the ophthalmic division of the trigeminal nerve and for midthoracic dermatomes, perhaps reflecting the centripetal distribution of the varicella rash. Zoster is derived from the Greek word for girdle. Approximately 10% of all patients with zoster develop postherpetic neuralgia; 50% of those over 60 years old do so. It is much more common after ophthalmic zoster than otherwise. Pain is described as steady with brief paroxysms in most patients.

Scarring, sensory loss, and exaggerated sensation of hyperesthesia, dysesthesia, and allodynia are quite common. Although the vesicular eruption may not have covered an entire dermatome, the pain does (Loeser, 1986).

Acyclovir is now the standard treatment, shown in double-blind studies to stop dissemination and speed healing in both normal and immunocompromised individuals. Ancillary treatments in the acute phase involve systemic triamcinolone, which reduces the duration of pain only in patients over 60. Oral prednisone reduces the likelihood of postherpetic neuralgia and shortens the duration of pain (Keczkes & Basheer, 1980). Nerve block has long been used for symptomatic treatment of acute herpes and postherpetic neuralgia. Most reports, all without controls, claim that peripheral, epidural, and sympathetic blocks in the acute phase provide prolonged pain relief if administered within the first 2 weeks. Nerve blocks, however, do not seem to lower the incidence of postherpetic neuralgia. One needs to remember, of course, the natural history of herpes zoster, namely, the very high likelihood of spontaneous pain resolution of patients under 50 and an increased likelihood of postherpetic neuralgia in patients over 60 years old. Many patients will have pain lasting for months but less than a year; very few have postherpetic pain lasting years.

Among conventional drug treatments, antidepressants (amitriptyline and nortriptyline) are useful in about 60% of patients. Topical capsaicin is about equally as effective. Anticonvulsant drugs such as carbamezapine and phenytoin are notable for their lack of efficacy in this condition, although they may prevent the lancinating pains (Watson, Evans, Watt & Birkett, 1988). Subcutaneous intralesional injection is advocated by Epstein (1973) using 2 mg of triamcinolone per milliliter of 0.25% bupivacaine. He claims nearly 100% acute pain relief and a reduced incidence of postherpetic neuralgia in his young patients. The treatment has no significant complications, and is simple and inexpensive (Raj, 1988).

Intercostal nerve blocks can relieve pain for 1 to 3 weeks.

Riopelle, Naraghi & Grush (1984) report that although inter-costal and stellate ganglion block, and lesional injections, provide relief of pain for a while, they do not appear to reduce the development of postherpetic neuralgia. They used stellate ganglion block with bupivacaine, local infiltration with bupivacaine and 0.2% triamcinolone, and intercostal block. Stellate ganglion block was used for pain above T4. Their 72 patients received 2 to 3 blocks each.

Raj (1988) also achieved good results for trigeminal zoster using stellate ganglion block. While intercostal or sympathetic block is a helpful adjunct in relieving the pain of this debilitating condition, no treatment, including nerve block, appears to reduce the incidence of the dreadful condition of postherpetic neuralgia in older patients. Neurolytic blocks rarely provide effective pain relief (nor does the pain of denervation respond well to narcotics, which should be used sparingly if at all). While nerve block can provide temporary pain relief, it is not necessarily a long-term management strategy because of tachyphylaxis associated with local anesthetics.

Technique of Intercostal Block

An intercostal nerve is the primary ramus of T1 to T11. A typical intercostal nerve has four branches: (1) the gray ramus communicans to the sympathetic chain; (2) the posterior cutaneous branch supplying paravertebral skin and muscles; (3) the lateral cutaneous division arising anterior to the midaxillary line; and (4) the anterior cutaneous branch that innervates the anterior midline. The nerve is accompanied by an intercostal vein and artery, which lie superior to the nerve in the inferior groove of each rib. Because of the proximity of these vessels, high blood levels of bupivacaine tend to accumulate after *multiple* intercostal blocks.

The most common site for block is at the angle of the rib. The patient is prone and a pillow placed under the abdomen to straighten the lumbar lordosis. If more than one nerve is to be blocked, it helps to mark the skin. This is done by first drawing a vertical line through the spinous processes. The ribs are at their most superficial 8 to 10 cm from this, depending on the size of the patient. A vertical line is drawn parallel to the first through this point. The inferior edge of the rib is palpated and a skin wheal raised.

For each intercostal nerve to be blocked, 5 ml of 0.25% bupivacaine with epinephrine is injected. A 1- to 1.5-in., 22-gauge needle is stuck vertically through the wheal after the skin is retracted superiorly. The retracted skin will help pull the needle off the rib inferiorly. Advancing 2 to 3 mm places the needle between the internal intercostal muscle and the intercostalis minimus where the nerve lies. It is important when walking the needle off the inferior edge of the rib to move the needle and syringe en bloc. If the syringe arcs superiorly while the needle point moves inferiorly, the anesthetic will be deposited too superficially.

The actual incidence of pneumothorax is rather low, although this is understandably the most considered complication of intercostal block. According to Moore and Bridenbaugh (1960) physicians in all stages of training performed over 10,000 intercostal blocks with an incidence of pneumothorax of 0.073%.

Low Back Pain

There are 8 million new physician visits annually for low back pain. While there are many causes for low back pain, three conditions account for the majority of cases, and nerve block has some role to play in them.

Mechanical problems, including myoligamentous strain and myodystonia from overuse, poor posture, and poor body mechanics, are more common than structural disease from arthritis. Herniated disk with true root compression follows. The L5 and S1 roots account for 90% of radiculopathies in the lower back. These three conditions need to be distinguished from each other.

Reasons to perform nerve block in back pain include the

development of muscle spasm no matter what the underlying disease is, and single lumbar root blockade for chronic back pain.

Degenerative Joint Disease

Vague back pain should not be dismissed as "arthritis," which has clear diagnostic criteria and objective findings. The pain is often worse on awakening after a night of immobility. Plain x rays disclose facet hypertrophy, joint sclerosis, osteophytosis, and other findings consistent with either destruction or growth of bone. Some specialists favor facet block in selected patients, but that technique is beyond the scope of this handbook.

Treatment of degenerative joint disease is usually with medication. Nerve block should be entertained, however, when there are excerbations of clinical symptoms associated with focal myodystonia. This is demonstrated by decreased forward bending and sharply circumscribed areas of myodystonia disclosed on palpation over the transverse processes or over the paravertebral musculature about 3 cm lateral to the spinous processes. Myofascial pain was discussed in Chapter 2.

Herniated Disk with Radiculopathy

As the term radiculopathy implies, low back pain from herniated nucleus pulposis (HNP) is associated with sensory symptoms in the leg. There are also diminished reflexes and specific weakness. Because sensory nerves are derived from two or more segments, motor signs are more reliable than sensory ones in the lower extremity, while the opposite holds true for the arm (Patten, 1977).

An L5 root is caused by herniation of the L4–L5 disk. Pain is felt in the back or lateral side of the side of the leg with radiation into the big toe. The knee-jerk is often reduced compared to the opposite side, and weakness of the extensor hallicus longus is the most reliable motor findings.

With the S1 root compressed, pain is perceived down the back of the thigh and into the little toe or lateral border of the foot. The ankle jerk is often diminished and there is difficulty with toe-walking. The L4 root, much less common, produces pain in a band from the lateral thigh wrapping medially down to the knee.

Many cases improve with conservative treatment of forced bed rest, analgesics, and antiinflammatory medication. The radicular pain often responds well to phenytoin or carbamezapine, although obviously in this case such chemical nerve suppression does nothing to address the cause of the pain. It may, however, relieve much agony until surgery can be done.

Because of the intense pain associated with HNP, there is often considerable myodystonia (reflex muscle spasm). It is sometimes not clear how much pain results from the spasm and how much from the disk itself. In this instance abolishing the muscular pain through trigger-point injection can easily sort out this problem. In this sense, nerve block is a diagnostic procedure in this circumstance.

Lumbar Myodystonia

As mentioned previously, this condition coexists as a reflex development from either arthritic degeneration of HNP. It can also exist by itself from the factors mentioned in Chapter 2. (See that chapter for the technique of field anesthesia.) It is a good adjuvant treatment to conservative therapy and muscle relaxers, and can distinguish how much pain arises from muscular structures and how much from nerve and bone.

Technique of Lumbar Somatic Nerve Block

Sometimes there are patients with chronic back and radicular pain who are not candidates for surgery for various reasons. In such patients, nerve block can provide pain relief that sometimes lasts for many months. It may also not be clear which root is causing the symptoms. In all these cases, block of a single nerve root can be used to arrive at the correct diagnosis.

The patient lies prone on a pillow to elevate the lumbar lordosis. A line is drawn horizontally across the superior aspect of the spinous process at the level to be blocked. Recall that at its superior aspect, the neural segment is always one above the vertebral segment. That is, the L4 root exists above the L5 vertebra and the T12 root above the L1 vertebra, and so forth.

Figure 4.4 shows the lateral location for needle insertion. An 8- to 10-cm needle is inserted perpendicularly to the skin surface 3 to 4 cm from the midline until it contacts the transverse process. This is usually 4 to 5 cm deep. The needle is then slightly withdrawn and aimed superiorly at 25° and inserted an additional 2 to 3 cm farther to contact the nerve. This frequently elicits parasthesias, and 8 to 10 ml of 0.25% bupivacaine is injected where this occurs. If no parasthesias are elicited, the bupivacaine is injected superior to the transverse process.

Anatomical facts to remember are that the transverse processes are short (3 to 4 cm from the vertebral lamina) and their average depth is 5 cm from the skin surface. The transverse processes of L4 and L5, however, are deeper. Last, because of the closeness of the L4 and L5 roots, both can be blocked by the same needle insertion at the superior border of the L4 transverse process. The L4 root is blocked by redirecting the needle superior to the transverse process, while the L5 root is blocked by redirecting the needle off its inferior border.

---→

FIGURE 4.4. Top: Landmarks for lumbar root injection. Bottom: The needle first hits the transverse process. Angulation 25° superiorly directs it off the bone and toward the spinal nerve, which lies 2 to 3 cm deeper. See text for further details. From Bridenbaugh, P. 1988. Neural Blockade and Pain Management, 2nd edition, p. 420. Copyright 1988 by Lippincott. Reprinted with permission.

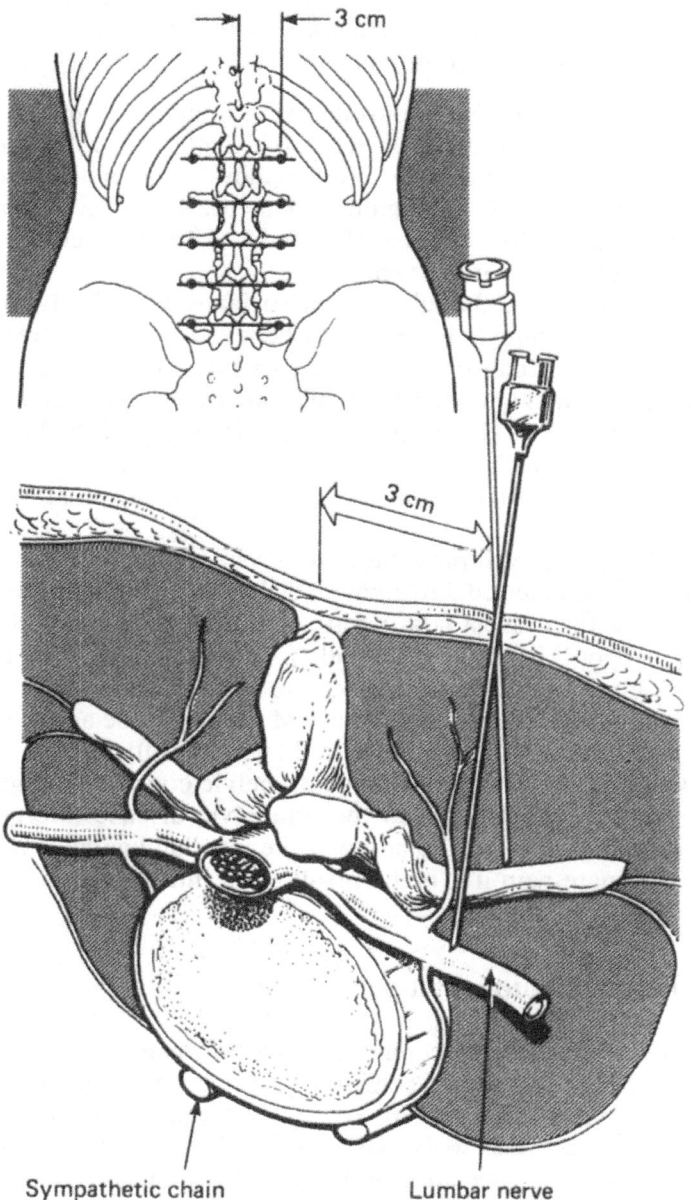

Sympathetic chain   Lumbar nerve

Meralgia Paresthetica: Block of the Lateral Femoral Cutaneous Nerve

Meralgia paraesthetica is burning pain, numbness, and tingling in the anterolateral aspect of the thigh, thought to be caused by entrapment of the lateral femoral cutaneous nerve as it passes through the inguinal ligament. It emerges from the fascia lata 1 to 2 cm medial to and 7 to 10 cm inferior to the anterior superior iliac spine.

The condition is thought to be associated with obesity or pregnancy. Although it is generally believed to be an entrapment, a specific cause is usually not found. The condition is common enough and the nerve easily accessible enough that nerve block is a rational treatment, certainly preferable to surgery, for which there are no good controlled studies. Weight loss is difficult to achieve in most patients and takes much time.

With the patient supine, the anterior iliac spine is palpated and a needle inserted 2 to 3 cm medial and 2 to 3 cm inferior to it. The firm fascia lata is felt soon after penetrating the skin; a "pop" is felt as the needle pierces it. Inject 10 ml of 0.25% bupivacaine fanwise along the superior–inferior axis; 2 ml of methylprednisolone (Depo-Medrol) may be added to the anesthetic (Miller, Munger & Powell, 1980).

Because the nerve has a long intrapelvic course, meralgia paresthetica can be caused by intrapelvic disease (uterus, prostate). A block of the nerve at the inguinal ligament will not eliminate pain if it is the result of an intrapelvic lesion.

Stellate Ganglion Sympathetic Block

There is considerable communication between the somatic roots and the sympathetic chain. One theory for the development of sympathetic hyperactivity is the ephaptic transmission or "cross talk" between sensory afferents and sympathetic efferents. One standard treatment regime is a series of three blocks at weekly intervals. Once therapeutic benefits

TABLE 4.2. Conditions that may be benefited by stellate ganglion block.

Pain
   Reflex sympathetic dystrophy, causalgia, sympathetically
      mediated pain
   Herpes zoster
   Paget's disease of bone
   Neoplasm
   Shoulder–hand syndrome, Sudeck's atrophy
   Cardiac pain
   Frostbite

Vascular Disorders
   Raynaud's phenomenon
   Occlusive arterial disease

---

have been established, the blocks can be spaced at increasing intervals in the hope that lasting relief occurs with each additional block. It may not be necessary to do a permanent neurolytic block or other surgical procedure in which the patient must trade permanent anesthesia for pain (Table 4.2).

Use of skilled occupational and physical therapists as an adjunct in treating reflex sympathetic dystrophy (RSD) is important, as are understanding psychological factors. Pain promotes emotional arousal, which in turn activates sympathetic efferents as well as increased muscle tone. The vicious cycle of continued pain, muscle spasm, and sympathetic hyperactivity can be broken through behavioral therapy, physical therapy, nerve block, and medical management. It is possible for the treating physician to wear several hats. Any pain, whether from soft tissue or nerve, can cause severe psychological disturbances (Table 4.3).

Injection of bupivacaine into the head and neck area, specifically the paravertebral fascia and stellate ganglion blocks, may produce adverse reactions similar to the systemic toxicity seen with large doses or unintentional intravascular or subarachnoid injection. These procedures therefore require

TABLE 4.3. Complications of stellate ganglion block.

Relatively Common
    Feeling a lump in the throat
    Hoarseness from recurrent laryngeal nerve anesthesia
    Temporary chest wall numbness

Uncommon
    Hematoma
    Pneumothorax
    Vertebral artery injection (immediate CNS complications)
    Intradural injection (slow onset of CNS effects)

considerable care. Pulse and blood pressure should be monitored during and after the procedure. Resuscitation equipment should be immediately available, and a stellate ganglion block should never be performed without an assistant.

There are several names for trauma-induced sympathetic pain: causalgia, RSD or sympathetically mediated pain. Whatever one chooses to call this, the name describes a constant burning pain in which gentle mechanical stimulation is excruciating (allodynia). That is, pain may be elicited by simply touching the skin, washing, or performing everyday tasks such as dressing or writing. If treatment to reduce the excessive sympathetic activity is not instituted early on, vasomotor, sudomotor, and trophic changes ensue after a few months. Vasomotor instability is evidenced by blanching, coldness, redness, and swelling of the digits. The digits may sweat profusely. The skin becomes thin and translucent, hair is lost, and sebaceous glands atrophy. Demineralization of bone is seen as a late sequela detected by a three-phase nuclear bone scan. Pain relief is dramatically achieved by sympathetic adrenergic blockade.

What causes RSD? (see Figure 4.5). Although there is not universal agreement, several factors clearly indicate that the pain is caused by *central* rather than peripheral dysfunction. The spinal wide dynamic range (WDR) neurons, which subserve pain, become highly responsive to gentle mechanical stimulation of A fibers after they are activated by C-fiber nociceptors. In other words, the initial trauma that activates the nociceptors also activates the WDR neurons in spinal cord. With time, sympathetic efferents to the mechanoreceptors result in a self-sustaining loop of mechanoreceptor afferents and sympathetic efferents sufficient to continuously stimulate the WDR neurons in spinal cord and their centripetal pain projections (Roberts, 1986).

Diagnosis and Therapy

The etiology of the initial trauma is of little importance because RSD follows a wide variety of initially painful disorders. Specific nerve injury is not required for the diagnosis. The inciting trauma of the peripheral tissue can be of any origin, such as crush, burn, fracture, or herpetic inflammation. Flexion extension injuries of the neck (whiplash) with or without radiculopathy often leads to later RSD.

Allodynia and hyperpathia are not crucial diagnostic signs. Response to sympathetic block or adrenergic blockers is the definitive diagnostic test. Emphasis in the acute phase is to prevent or minimize the sensitization of the WDR neurons by reducing the nociceptor input. This can be achieved by methods ranging from antiinflammatory agents to triggerpoint injections and peripheral nerve block. Once chronic pain develops, however, all treatments lose their effectiveness.

Sympathetic block of the stellate ganglion relieves RSD by removing the self-sustaining sympathetic excitation to the A-fiber mechanoreceptors. This in turn results in dysfacilitation of the WDR neurons and a reduction in the burning pain and allodynia associated with it. Pain relief is usually quite prolonged, particularly if it is done early in the course of RSD (Bonica, 1970). Because of the long-lasting relief that sympathetic blocks give, it is probably the postganglionic neurons that excite the relevant afferents. The important point is that this condition should be treated as soon as it is diagnosed.

Technique and Anatomy

Although the sympathetic preganglionic fibers of the head, neck, and arm are formed by the T1 to T6 segments, they converge anterior to the neck of the first rib where the first thoracic and inferior cervical ganglia may fuse to form the stellate ganglion. The anatomy of the cervical sympathetic

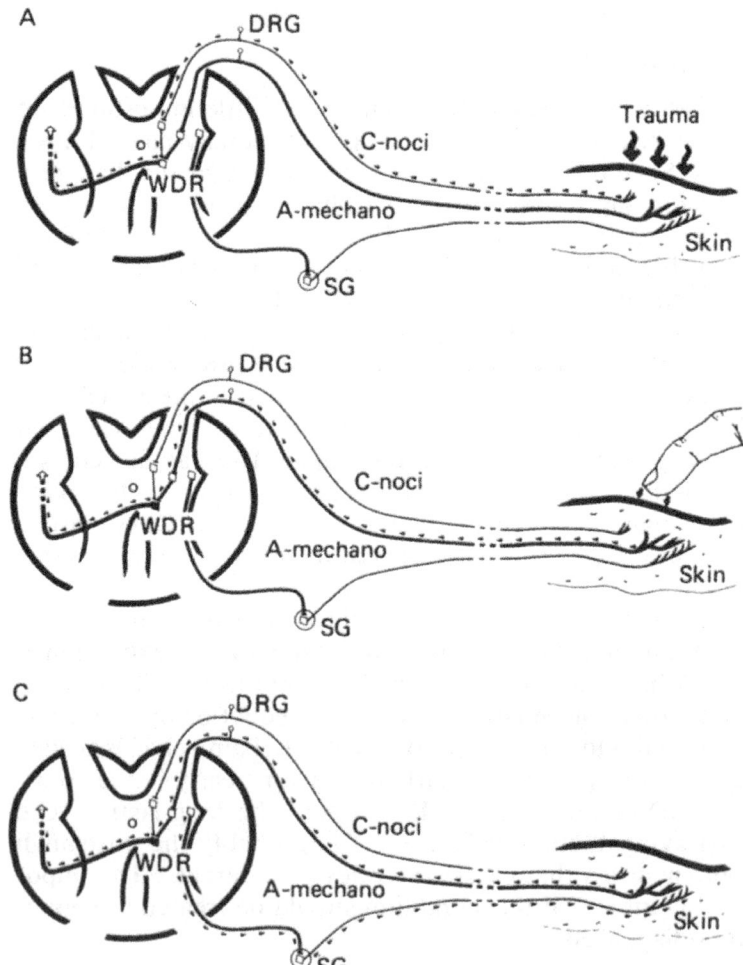

chain, however, is quite variable, and for this reason a large volume of anesthetic is required to achieve good results. Fifteen to 20 ml of 0.25% bupivacaine injected in front of the C6 transverse process will usually extend in front of the prevertebral fascia at least down to T4. Leriche first developed this paratracheal approach in 1934 as a way to avoid the risk of pneumothorax inherent in injecting at the first rib.

The physician stands on the side to be blocked. Bilateral block should never be done at the same time. The patient is supine and the neck extended to stretch the esophagus away from the transverse process on the left side. A small neck roll is useful. With adequate information and preparation, most patients hold quite still and sandbags or bolsters to prevent head rotation are rarely needed.

The C6 transverse process, or Chassaignac's tubercle, is the landmark. It lies below the cricoid cartilage as seen in Figure 4.6. The carotid artery is retracted laterally and the trachea pushed to the midline. A 1.5-in., 21-gauge needle is attached to a 20-ml syringe of 0.25% bupivacaine by an extension tube. The needle is inserted paramedial at the level of the cricoid cartilage until it hits bone. At this point it is resting on the C6 transverse process. The palpating fingers hold their position while the right hand withdraws the needle 2 mm and holds it fixed in that position.

The assistant aspirates both before and after rotating the

FIGURE 4.5. Physiological development self-sustaining reflex loop in sympathetic dystrophy. A. Through the C nociceptors, the initial trauma sensitizes the wide dynamic range (WDR) neurons, whose axons ascend to higher pain centers. B. The sensitized WDR neurons now respond to the large-diameter A mechanoreceptors, activated by light touch and other mechanical stimulation. This produces allodynia. C. The same WDR neurons again respond to A-mechanoreceptor activity in the absence of touch, this time being activated by sympathetic efferents. From Roberts, W. J. 1986. "A Hypothesis on the Psychological Basis for Causalgia and Related Pains", p. 300, in Pain, 24. Copyright 1986 by Elsevier. Reprinted with permission.

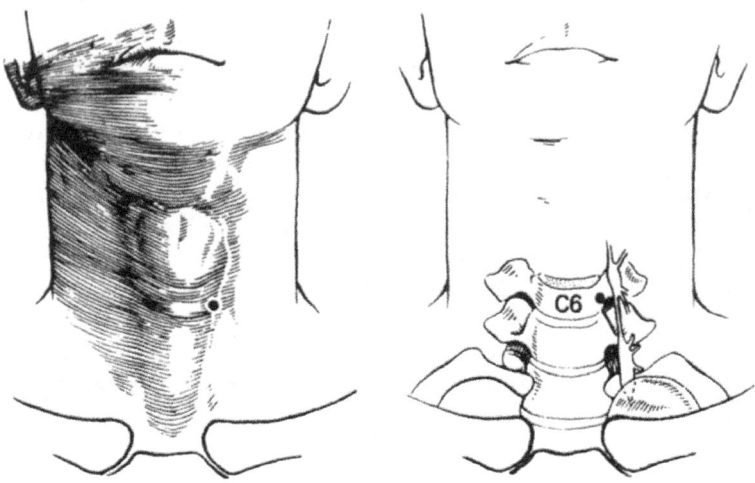

FIGURE 4.6. The cricoid cartilage is the landmark for stellate ganglion block. The stellate ganglion lies just anterior to this. From Cousins, M. J. 1988. "Introduction to Acute and Chronic Pain: Implications for Neural Blockade", p. 481, in Neural Blockade, 2nd edition, Cousins & Bridenbaugh (eds.). Copyright 1988 by Lippincott. Reprinted with permission.

needle 90°. If aspiration is negative for blood and cerebrospinal fluid (CSF), a test dose of 2 ml is injected. If the patient feels nothing and no untoward effects develop, the remaining volume is injected. There should be no resistance at all. If there is, the needle is either in periosteum or prevertebral muscle. Under no circumstances should injection be performed if blood enters the syringe, because even a few milliliters injected into the vertebral artery can result in convulsions, cortical blindness, or other neurological loss. There should also be no resistance to the needle until it hits bone. If resistance is felt, it is usually from the prevertebral fascia and muscles connecting the transverse processes, an indication that the needle penetration is too close to the midline. In too medial a location, the needle may enter a dural cuff that surrounds the cervical nerve roots. If so, CSF may enter the syringe on aspiration although a positive aspiration is not always the case. Injection into the dural sheath will result in spinal anesthesia.

A successful block produces Horner's syndrome: ptosis, miosis, and conjunctival flushing. The arm will become warm. Blood pressure and pulse should be monitored before, during, and after the procedure. The patient should stay recumbent and be observed for 30 minutes after the procedure. It is quite common to feel a lump in the throat or be temporarily hoarse following this procedure. In addition to judging the immediate effects, patients should be instructed to keep a pain diary, rating the severity of pain and frequency of paroxysms for the week following the block.

5 —
Cognitive Aspects of Pain

Because there are many facets in pain treatment and research, much data on many axes could be collected for each
patient. The bulk of such activity is academic, however. The
practical question should be what is useful.

Rudy, Turk and Brena (1988) looked at the differential
utility of medical procedures in the assessment of pain patients and asked how to weigh and integrate the findings.
They found substantial agreement regarding the utility of 18
examination and diagnostic procedures. Only 6 of these 18,
however, were ranked in the top third of usefulness by 50%
or more of the physicians sampled. Tables 5.1 and 5.2 show
that, despite technical advances, the physical examination
remains the most useful procedure.

TABLE 5.1. Linear weights for 18 medical procedures
in pain assessment.[a]

Weight[b]	Medical procedure
0.394	Neurologic examination
0.364	Gait and posture
0.354	Spine mobility
0.339	Muscular function (tone, mass, strength)
0.317	Soft-tissue exam
0.301	Mobility of weight-bearing joints
0.260	Mobility of non-weight-bearing joints
0.239	Plain film
0.219	CT scan
0.196	Electromyography
0.166	Contrast radiography
0.134	Internal medicine examination
0.107	Nuclear medicine
0.082	Lab tests (other than blood)
0.071	Blood count
0.039	Thermography
0.009	Electroencephalography
0.007	Electrocardiography

[a]From Rudy, Turk and Brena (1988).
[b]Weights are standardized to sum to 1.00 when
squared.

TABLE 5.2. Relevance of 18 medical procedures in pain assessment.[a]

Percentage of cases rated as relevant	Procedure
100	Soft-tissue examination
98	Neurological examination
98	Gait and posture
97	Muscular function
96	Spinal mobility
90	Mobility of weight-bearing joints
88	Mobility of non-weight-bearing joints
87	Plain film
84	Thermography
65	Electromyography
64	Internal medicine examination
56	CT scan
36	Lab tests (other than blood)
33	Blood count
32	Contrast radiography
20	Nuclear medicine
15	Electrocardiography
10	Electroencephalography

[a]From Rudy, Turk and Brena (1988).

Rudy et al. made no mention of psychological factors, which is what I want to consider briefly in this last chapter. The physician must, after all, address the patient's "total pain."

Some may say that they have no experience or interest in psychological analysis or cognitive evaluation, but such an objection is simply throwing up one's hands. Such naysayers are likely to respond by pumping yet more pills at patients and then blaming them for not getting better. I will focus on assessments and interventions that are practical, easily available, and can influence the clinical situation.

We are accustomed to thinking, erroneously, that machine tests are "objective" and thus more accurate than any subjective self-reporting. Yet pain involves a wide variety of physiological, psychological, and environmental factors. Because "diagnosis" means "through knowledge," the physician needs knowledge of the patient's psychological makeup and characteristic coping style to make effective interventions. The approach of framing something as simple as the MMPI in terms of "this test will help me understand how you think and cope with illness" puts it in a positive light and actively engages the patient in his own treatment.

As I mentioned in Chapter 1, neurotic features are a consequence and not a cause of pain. That this is so is shown by MMPI studies in which elevations of the neurotic triad (the first three scales) decrease when chronic pain is relieved. Although there is still an unfortunate tendency to dichotomize patients into organic versus functional, organic patients do, with time, undergo emotional and psychological changes. Our purpose here is not so much to try to distinguish between organic and psychogenic pain but rather to look at those psychological and emotional factors that accompany pain and how understanding them can help treatment. Such assessment helps the physician predict who will respond to certain kinds of treatment, who is likely to fail, and which patients are receptive to exploring psychological factors compared to those who demand a mechanistic approach and shun all attempts to investigate emotional factors.

There are patients, of course, in whom the psychological approach is completely hopeless. Such patients have a constricted affect, are unable to verbalize their feelings, and have enormous difficulty perceiving a connection between bodily sensations and emotional feelings. The term used to describe this state is alexithymia, meaning "no words for feelings" (Cytowic, 1985; Lesser, 1985).

Factors That Modulate Pain

The modulation of pain by nonpainful events is well accepted (Wall, 1976), although the classical view of pain was rather simplistic: namely, that a mechanistic, anatomical pathway produced sensation that could be related to a physical event while later mental processes (learning, emotion, and memory) could exaggerate or ignore the mechanistic report sent to the brain. In the classical view the presence of a direct projection from periphery to the brain was completely accepted. Small myelinated and unmyelinated fibers were conceived to terminate on spinal cells whose axons projected to ventrolateral white matter, thalamus, and so forth. As Wall points out, the entire theory was based on only two facts: the requirement of small-diameter peripheral nerve fibers to perceive pain, and the analgesia produced by sectioning ventrolateral white tracts in the cord. "All the rest was speculation, implication and guesswork."

A number of clinical observations indicates that this conception is too simplistic. Referred pain, for example, proves that convergence from uninjured tissue does modulate the perception of pain. Indeed the gate theory depends on such convergence as well as descending controls from brain stem and cortex. Certainly no biological system is driven by excitation alone, uncountered by feedback and feed-forward forces. The pain system is therefore like any other biological system in this regard. One conclusion regarding convergence is that one should not expect that cutting nerves or pain tracts will abolish pain permanently, because there are ancillary routes for transmission.

I have already said a lot about placebos. Much can also be achieved by paying attention to factors that *modulate* pain (see Table 5.3). For example, carefully explaining the mechanism of pain reduces anxiety, supports the therapeutic relationship, and boosts morale. Twycross (1984) points out that "ignoring mental and social factors may result in otherwise relievable pain remaining intractable." Giving the patient a sense of control is important. Ninety-seven ICU patients who were told what to expect following surgery, how to relax by deep breathing, and how to move so they would be most comfortable postoperatively, required half the analgesia of the control group and were discharged 3 days earlier. But before such teaching can be done, the phy-

TABLE 5.3. Factors affecting pain threshold.[a]

Lowers threshold	Raises threshold
Discomfort	Relief of symptoms
Insomnia	Sleep
Fatigue	Rest
Anxiety	Sympathy
Fear	Understanding
Anger	Companionship
Sadness	Diversion
Depression	Reduction of anxiety
Boredom	Elevation of mood
Introversion	Analgesics
Mental isolation	Anxiolytics
Social abandonment	Antidepressants

[a]From Twycross (1984).

sician must understand the nonmechanistic aspects of the patient's pain perception.

It is particularly unfortunate that physicians have little reference to patients with chronic pain, which is a situation rather than a transient event that seems to have no end, often gets worse than better, lacks any meaning, and often expands to occupy all the patient's attention. This further isolates him from social and work spheres.

Patients often put on a good face for the doctor for reasons not entirely clear. A true picture of the pain, rather than focusing on the PQRST factors (provocation, quality, radiation, severity, time), is gained by probing into larger issues such as when is the last time you had a vacation, what are you doing around the house, when is the last time you socialized, etc. This strengthens the therapeutic relationship by showing concern for humanistic areas and may be the first step in taking the focus away from pain, opening the patient up and getting him out of himself.

Psychological diversions do more than just pass the time. They actually diminish pain and their benefit should not be

TABLE 5.4. Psychological and related
methods of pain control.[a]

Distraction	Massage
Imagery	Heat
Relaxation	Pressure
Biofeedback	TENS
Hypnosis	Acupuncture

[a]From Twycross (1984).

forgotton. Pain is worse when it occupies the patient's
whole attention (Table 5.4).

Most pain can eventually be controlled. Regarding an ultimate goal of "total pain relief," one paradoxically finds
greater success in achieving stepwise relief. Goals need to
be clearly thought out. Some pain responds more readily
than other. The first target should be an undisturbed night's
sleep. To awaken refreshed from a sound night's sleep after
months or weeks of agony is not only refreshing but quite
moralizing and not to be underestimated. One can next aim
for freedom from pain while resting in the bed or chair during the day. Freedom from pain on movement or during
daily activities is the final goal. The former is always eventually possible, but the latter is not; one needs to maintain a
realistic outlook. The physician should not underestimate
the encouragement achieved by relief at night and when
resting during the day. This produces a whole new psychol-
ogy and gives new hope.

The Minnesota Multiphasic Personality Inventory (MMPI)

Various empirically derived (MMPI) profiles have been used
for differential diagnosis, prediction of treatment outcome,
and in patient–treatment matching.

Costello et al. (1987) labeled their four profile types P, A, I, and N. The P-sychopathological types have all scales elevated and are extreme in their endorsement of physical symptoms and psychological distress. They have poor education, high unemployment, and low income. The A-types have a conversion V on the triad scales (scales 1, 2, and 3) and no unique demographic correlates. I-Types have elevations of the neurotic scales and no others, and appear to be the most physically infirm with multiple surgeries and hospitalizations. They usually do not improve with treatment but do benefit psychologically. N-types are N"ormal" with no elevations except perhaps the K scale. N-types are moderate in their claims of ill health, and often are better educated, are employed, and appear to respond well to treatment.

Love and Peck (1987) review the use of the MMPI as a predictor for treatment of low back pain but point out that although the concept of a psychological etiology of chronic back pain has failed, it continues to be widely used. Indeed the special Low Back (LB) scale by Hanvick (1951) and the dorsal (DOR) scale by Pichot have not been replicated (Calsyn, Louks & Freeman, 1976). What the MMPI *can* do is distinguish between different types of psychological responses to pain. This is just further evidence against the functional versus organic dichotomy.

It is true that many patients with chronic pain show the conversion V profile of elevated 1 and 3 (Hs and Hy) scales and a slightly lower 2 (D) scale. This conversion triad reflects a defensive personality unaware of psychological conflict who expresses such conflicts via physical symptoms. While this personality is found in many pain patients, it is also found in nonpain patients, and the mistake is in suggesting that it represents a psychogenic cause rather than *the response* to the problem. Love and Peck reviewed studies that seriously question the usefulness of the conversion V concept. On close examination of individual MMPI profiles, it turns out that patients often have elevated 1 and 3 scales because they do appropriately endorse items that are relevant to their actual physical condition.

Brena et al. (1980; Chapman & Brena, 1982) studied responses to spinal nerve block, and while they did find objective organic signs and conversion V profiles there was no predictive relationship between the conversion V scores and response to treatment. Moreover their studies, and others, show that conversion V profiles are quite common and that their presence does not rule out success of various treatments. My opinion is that the MMPI is useful for the physician to better understand the psychological makeup and characteristic coping style of individual patients. Finding the so-called P type of Costello makes me more sanguine that I will make a significant difference in that patient's functioning.

Chapman and Brena (1982) investigated response to nerve block in low back patients with "learned helplessness," measured by dependence on narcotic analgesics, low activity levels, and elevated MMPI scales 1, 2, and 3. They treated them with both bupivacaine and placebo saline injections. Greater reduction in subjective pain was found for both types of blocks in patients who had low levels of pain behavior, were divorced, and had no pending disability claims. Chapman and Brena concluded that chronic pain patients who were fixed in their focus of pain and had high pain behavior and low responsibilities are less likely to respond favorably to nerve block, and that these factors need to be considered in finding a strategy to reduce their helplessness.

The MMPI has also been used in headache. Williams et al. (1986) reviewed the individualized analysis of the MMPI for treatment of headache. Psychological factors have long been assumed to be important in headache of various types, particularly migraine. For example, migraneurs are stereotyped as ambitious, perfectionistic, compulsive, rigid, resentful, and unable to express aggressive feelings constructively, whereas tension headache patients are prone to worry, depression, and anxiety and are characteristically tense and may have psychosexual conflicts.

The MMPI is useful in the differential diagnosis of headache. According to several studies, migraine and cluster

TABLE 5.5. MMPI classification of Kudrow–Sutkus headache groups.[a]

Group	Type of headache	Classification criteria of scales 1, 2, and 3
Females	Migraine and cluster	T < 65 for scales 1 and 2
	Tension and mixed	65 < T > 70 for scales 2 and 3
	Posttraumatic and psychogenic	T > 70 for 2 or more scales
Males	Migraine and cluster	T < 70 for scales 2 and 3
	Tension and mixed	T > 70 for 2 or more scales
	Posttraumatic and psychogenic	T > 75 for all scales

[a]From Kudrow & Sutkus (1979).

types consistently have considerably less psychological distress than either muscle contraction or mixed headaches. Posttraumatic and psychogenic headaches are the most distressed within the headache population. The posttraumatic type is probably so because of actual physical symptoms, which are often not believed by their physicians, attorneys, compensation boards, and families (as I mentioned earlier).

Kudrow and Sutkus (1979) have made a most useful grouping according to scales 1, 2, and 3 of the MMPI. Their three groups are migraine and cluster, muscle contraction and mixed headaches, and posttraumatic and psychogenic. The differences between the diagnostic criteria in male and female groups are shown in Table 5.5.

This study, and later ones that validated it, show a continuum of psychological distress with a χ^2 prediction accuracy exceeding 0.001. Migraine and cluster patients (the least neurotic) have a mild degree of worry and somatization whereas the posttraumatic and conversion headaches have the most "neurotic looking" profiles. This does not mean that these headaches are purely psychogenic, as was mentioned. It is rather interesting and unexpected that cluster headache patients are the least disturbed psychologically, given how debilitating the headaches are. Patients have been known to commit suicide because of them.

The MMPI has also been used to predict treatment outcome. However, such studies are few in number, making it difficult to reach definitive conclusions. Multivariate analysis of peak scale scores for successful versus unsuccessful participants in a biofeedback relaxation program showed significant relationships. Unsuccessful patients had a conversion V profile, whereas successful patients had peak scores for scales 2 and 0. The authors (Werder et al., 1981) suggested that successful patients were more aware of their internal discomfort.

Very little literature exists on using the MMPI or similar psychometric instruments in matching patients with particular treatments. Williams et al. (1986) provides a review and some suggestions. Those patients who have little discernible psychological difficultly, both by history and on psychometric tests, make good candidates for biofeedback or relaxation training, particularly if their lifestyles favor a nondrug approach. Patients with clinical and psychometric evidence of distress may benefit from individualized goal-directed therapy. Patients with more severe distress, particularly with high scales 8 and 9, may benefit from adding a major tranquilizer.

In conclusion, MMPI studies show that psychopathology is not distributed across diagnostic headache groups, although headache patients are more disturbed than nonheadache controls. In ascending order of disturbance, one finds migraine, cluster, tension, mixed, and posttraumatic headaches.

Psychological Contributions to Pain

A number of investigators have shown there are cultural determinants to the perception of pain and pain tolerance. These reflect different ethnic attitudes toward pain. For example, Old Americans (Puritans) are stoic whereas Jews and

Italians are more vociferous and openly seek support and sympathy. Children are deeply influenced by parental attitudes and carry these into adulthood. Context also matters. Soldiers wounded in battle rarely complain of pain whereas civilians with similar injuries respond with great distress.

Attention, anxiety, and distraction are also factors. If a patient's attention is focused on a potentially painful experience, he will perceive that pain more intensely than he otherwise would. The mere anticipation of pain is sufficient to raise the level of anxiety and therefore the level of perceived pain. The more control a patient feels he has, then the less disturbing will the pain be. For this reason, patients about to undergo procedures do best if given detailed information about what will happen, what to expect, and what they can do to mitigate the unpleasantness (e.g., relaxation, deep breathing, requesting p.r.n. medication). Everything that can be done to provide the patient with a sense of control is helpful.

Finally, relaxation and meditation based on various religious practices do result in striking physiological changes (decreased muscle tone, lowered blood pressure and respiration). In turn, this does produce significant reductions of pain (Benson, Pomeranz & Katz, 1984).

Appendix A

Common CPT–4 Codes for Nerve Block and Trigger-Point Injection

64405	Injection, anesthetic agent, greater occipital nerve
64413	Cervical plexus
64420	Intercostal nerve, single
64440	Paravertebral nerve, single
64441	Paravertebral nerve, multiple
64450	Peripheral nerve or branch
64510	Stellate ganglion block
20550	Injection, anesthetic agent, tendon sheath, ligament or trigger point

Appendix B

Common ICD–9 Diagnoses for Nerve Block and Trigger-Point Injection (consult the ICD–9 manual for fourth digit depending on clinical circumstance)

Neural Disorders

353.x	Nerve root and plexus disorders
354.x	Nerve lesion, upper extremity (e.g., carpal tunnel syndrome, 3540
3544	Causalgia
355.x	Nerve lesion, lower extremity
3551	Meralgia paresthetica
356.x	Hereditary and idiopathic peripheral neuropathy
357.x	Inflammatory and toxic neuropathy
3370	Autonomic neuropathy (sympathetic dystrophy)

Injuries (codes 953–957)

955	Injury, peripheral nerve
951	Injury, cranial nerve
9570	Injury, superficial nerves of head and neck

Myoligamentous Disorders

(An enthesopathy is a disorder of peripheral ligaments or muscular attachments.)

7201	Spinal enthesopathy
726.x	Peripheral enthesopathy
721	Spondylosis and allied disorders (strains and sprains)
7242	Low back pain
7231	Neck pain
840	Myoligamentous strain, brachial or cervical
846	Myoligamentous strain, lumbar

References

Abram, S.E., Anderson, R.A., Maitra-D'Cruze, A.M. 1981. Factors predicting short-term outcome of nerve blocks in the management of chronic pain. Pain 10:323–320.

American College of Physicians, Health and Public Policy Committee. 1983. Drug therapy for severe chronic pain in terminal illness. Ann. Intern. Med. 99:870–873.

Angell, M. 1982. The quality of mercy. N. Engl. J. Med. 306:98–99.

Beals, R.K., Hickman, N.W. 1972. Industrial injuries of the back and extremities. J. Bone Joint Surg. 54A:1593–1611.

Beecher, H.K. 1955. The powerful placebo. JAMA 159:1602–1606.

Benson, H., Pomeranz, B., Katz, I. 1984. The relaxation response and pain. In: Wall, P.D., Melzack R., eds. Textbook of Pain. Edinburgh: Churchill Livingstone.

Bonica, J.J. 1953. The management of Pain. Philadelphia: Lea & Febiger.

Bonica, J.J. 1970. Causalgia and other reflex sympathetic dystrophies. In: Bonica, J.J., et al., eds. Advances in Pain Research and Therapy, Vol. 3, pp. 141–166. New York: Raven Press.

Bonica, J.J. 1988. Neural blockade in the multidisciplinary pain clinic. In: Cousins, M.J., Bridenbaugh, P.O., eds. Neural Blockade, 2nd Ed., pp. 1119–1138. Philadelphia: Lipincott.

Brena, S.F. 1985. Nerve blocks and chronic pain states—an update. Postgrad. Med. 78(4):62–71.

Brena, S.F., Wolf, S.L., Chapman, S.L., Hamonds, W.D. 1980. Chronic back pain: electromyographic, motion and behavioral assessments following sympathetic nerve blocks and placebos. Pain 8:1–10.

Calsyn, D.A., Louks, J., Freeman, C.W. 1976. The use of the MMPI with chronic low back pain patients with a mixed diagnosis. J. Clin. Psychol. 32:532–536.

Catchlove, S.L., Cohen, K. 1982. Effects of a directive return to work approach in the treatment of workmen's compensation patients with chronic pain. Pain 14:181–191.

Chapman, S.L., Brena, S.F. 1982. Learned helplessness and responses to nerve blocks in chronic low back pain patients. Pain 14:355–364.

Charap, A.D. 1978. The knowledge, attitudes, and experience of medical personnel treating pain in the terminally ill. Mt Sinai J Med. (NY) 45:561–580.

Colvin, D.F., Bettinger, R., Knapp, R., Pawlicki, R., Zimmerman, J. 1980. Characteristics of patients with chronic pain. S. Med. J. 73(8):1020–1023.

Costello, R.M., Hulsey, T.L., Schoenfeld, L.S., Samamurthy, S. 1987. P-A-I-N: a four-cluster MMPI typology for chronic pain. Pain 30:199–209.

Cousins, M.J. 1988. Introduction to acute and chronic pain: Implications for neural blockade. In: Cousins, M.J., Bridenbaugh, P.O., eds. Neural Blockade, 2nd Ed., pp. 739–752. Philadelphia: Lippincott.

Cytowic, R.E. 1985. Alexithymia—or stupidity? N. Engl. J. Med. 313:53.

Cytowic, R.E., Stump, D.A., Larned, D.C. 1988. Closed head trauma: somatic, ophthalmic and cognitive impairments in non-hospitalized patients. In: Whitaker, H.A., ed. Neuropsychologic Studies of Nonfocal Brain Damage: Dementia and Trauma, pp. 226–265. New York: Springer-Verlag.

Dworkin, R.H., Handlin, D.S., Richlin, D.M., Brand, L., Vannucci, C. 1985. Unraveling the effects of compensation, litigation and employment on treatment response in chronic pain. Pain 23:49–59.

Egbert, L.D., Battit, G.E., Welch, C.E., Bartlett, M.K. 1964. Reduction of postoperative pain by encouragement and instruction of patients—a study of doctor–patient rapport. N. Engl. J. Med. 270:825–827.

Epstein, E. 1973. Intralesional triamcinolone therapy in herpes zoster and postzoster neuralgia. Eye Nose Throat J. 52:61.

Evans, F.J. 1974. The placebo response in pain reduction. Adv. Neurol. 4:289–296.

Fine, P.G., Melano, R., Hare, B.D. 1988. The effects of myofascial trigger point injection are naloxone reversible. Pain 32:15–20.

Foley, K.M. 1985. The treatment of cancer pain. N. Engl. J. Med. 313(2):84–95.

Gilroy, J., Meyer, J.S. 1975. Medical Neurology, 2nd Ed. New York: Macmillan.

Goodwin, J.S., Goodwin J.M., Vogel, A.V. 1979. Knowledge and use of placebos by house officers and nurses. Ann. Intern. Med. 91:106–110.

Hanvick, L.J., MMPI profiles in patients with low back pain. 1951. J. Consult. Clin. Psychol. 15:350–353

Keczkes, K., Basheer, A.M. 1980. Do corticosteroids prevent post herpetic neuralgia? Br. J. Dermatol. 102:551–555.

Kelly, R.E. 1981. The post-traumatic syndrome. J. R. Soc. Med. 74:242–245.

Kelly, R.E., Smith, B.N. 1981. Post-traumatic syndrome: another myth discredited. J. R. Soc. Med. 74:275–277.

Khoury, G., Varga, C.A. 1988. Does frequency of utilization of nerve blocks in pain clinics vary with the specialty of the director? Pain 33:265.

Kraus, H. 1970. Clinical treatment of back and neck pain. New York: McGraw-Hill.

Kudrow, L., Sutkus, B.J. 1979. MMPI pattern specificity in primary headache disorders. Headache 19:18–24.

Leavitt, F., Sweet, J.J. 1986. Characteristics and frequency of malingering among patients with low back pain. Pain 25:357–364.

Lesser, I.M. 1985. Alexithymia. N. Engl. J. Med. 312:690–692.

Levine, J.D., Gordon, N.C., Fields, H.L. 1978. The mechanism of placebo analgesia. Lancet ii:654–657.

Loeser, J.D. 1986. Herpes Zoster and postherpetic neuralgia. Pain 25:149–164.

Love, A.W., Peck, C.L. 1987. The MMPI and psychological factors in chronic low back pain: a review. Pain 28:1–12.

Marks, R.M., Sachar, E.J. 1973. Undertreatment of medical inpatients with narcotic analgesics. Ann. Intern. Med. 78:173–181.

Mayer, D.J., Price, D.D. 1976. Central nervous system mechanisms of analgesia. Pain 2:379–404.

Mayer, T.G. 1983. Rehabilitation of the patient with spinal pain. Orthop. Clin. North Am. 14:623–637.

McCain, G.A., Scudds, R.A. 1988. The concept of primary fibromyalgia (fibrositis): clinical value, relation and significance to other chronic musculoskeletal pain syndromes. Pain 33:273–287.

McGivey, W.T., Crooks, G.M., eds. 1984. The care of patients with severe chronic pain in terminal illness. JAMA 251:1182–1188.

Melzack, R. 1973. The puzzle of pain. New York: Basic Books.

Melzack, R. 1981. Myofascial trigger points: relation to acupuncture and mechanisms of pain. Arch. Phys. Med. Rehabil. 62:114–117.

Melzack, R. 1988. Psychological aspects of pain: implications for neural blockade, In: Cousins, M.J., Bridenbaugh, P.O., eds. Neural Blockade, pp. 845–859. Philadelphia: Lippincott.

Mendelson, G. 1982. Not 'cured by a verdict:' effect of legal settlement on compensation claimants. Med. J. Aust. 2:132–134.

Mendelson, G. 1984. Compensation, pain complaints, and psychological disturbances. Pain 20:169.

Merskey, H., ed. 1986. Classification of chronic pain. Description of chronic pain syndromes and definitions of pain terms. Pain 3(Suppl.):1.

Merskey, H., Boyd, D. 1978. Emotional adjustment and chronic pain. Pain 5:173–178.

Miller, R.D., Munger, W.L., Powell, P.E. 1980. Chronic pain and local anethetic neural blockade. In: Cousins, M.J., Bridenbaugh, P.O., eds. Neural Blockade, pp. 616–636. Philadelphia: Lippincott.

Moore, D.C., Bridenbaugh, L.D. 1960. Pneumothorax: its incidence following intercostal nerve block. JAMA 174:842.

Patten, J. 1977. Neurological differential diagnosis. New York: Springer-Verlag.

Peck, C.J., Fordyce, W.E., Black, R.G. 1978. The effect of the pendency of claims for compensation upon behavior indicative of pain. Wash. Law Rev. 53:251–278.

Porter, J., Jick, H. 1980 Addiction rare in patients treated with narcotics. N. Engl. J. Med. 302:123.

Raj. P.P. 1988. Prognostic and therapeutic local anesthetic blockade, In: Cousins, M.J., Bridenbaugh, P.O., eds. Neural Blockade, 2nd ed., pp. 899–ff. Philadelphia: Lippincott.

Reuler, J.B., Girard, D.E., Nardone, D.A. 1980. The chronic pain syndrome: misconceptions and management. Ann. Intern. Med. 93:588–596.

Riopelle, A.M., Naraghi, M., Grush, K.P. 1984. Chronic neuralgia incidence following local anesthetic therapy for herpes zoster. Arch. Dermatol. 120:747–750.

Roberts, W.J. 1986. A hypothesis on the physiological basis for causalgia and related pains. Pain 24:297–311.

Rudy, T.E., Turk, D.C., Brena, S.F. 1988. Differential utility of medical procedures in the assessment of chronic pain patients. Pain 34:53–60.

Saunders, C.M. 1967. The Management of Terminal Illness. London: Edward Arnold.

Simons, D.G. 1975. Special review, muscle pain syndromes. Part I. Am. J. Phys. Med. 54:289–311. Part II. Am. J. Phys. Med. 55:15–42.

Sriwatanakul, K., Weiss, O.F., Alloza, J.L., Kelvie, W., Weintraub, M., Lasagna, L. 1983. Analysis of narcotic analgesic useage in the treatment of postoperative pain. JAMA 250:926–1292.

Sternbach, R.A. 1974. Pain Patients: Traits and Treatment. New York: Academic Press.

Sternbach, R.A. 1976. Psychological factors in pain. In: Bonica, J.J., Albe-Fessard, D., eds. Advances in Pain Research and Therapy, Vol. 1, pp. 293–299. New York: Raven Press.

Travell, J. 1976. Myofascial trigger points: clinical view. In: Bonica, J.J., Albe-Fessard, D., eds. Advances in Pain Research and Therapy, Vol. 1, pp. 919–926. New York: Raven Press.

Travell, J.G., Simons, D.G. 1983. Myofascial Pain and Dysfunction: The Trigger Point Manual. Baltimore: Williams & Wilkins.

Twycross, R.G. 1984. Control of pain. J.R. Coll. Physicians Lond. London 18(1):32–39.

Twycross, R.G., Fairfield, S. 1982. Pain in far-advanced cancer. Pain 14:303–310.

Viano, D.C. 1988. Cause and control of automotive trauma. Bull. N. Y. Acad. Med. 54(5):376–421.

Wall, P.D. 1976. Modulation of pain by nonpainful events. In: Bonica, J.J., Albe-Fessard, D., eds. Advances in Pain Research and Therapy, Vol. 1. New York: Raven Press.

Watson, C.P.N., Evans, R.J., Watt, V.R., Birkett, N. 1988. Post herpetic neuralgia: 208 cases. Pain 35:289–297.

Weighill, V.E. 1983. 'Compensation neurosis:' a review of the literature. J. Psychosom. Res. 27:97–104.

Werder, D.S., Sargent, J.D., Coynes, L. 1981. MMPI profiles of headache patients using self-regulation to control headache activity. Headache 21:164–169.

Williams, D.A., Thorn, B.E. 1989. An empirical assessment of pain beliefs. Pain 36:351–358.

Williams, D.E., Thompson, J.K., Haber, J.D., Raczyniski, J.M. 1986. MMPI and headache: a special focus on differential diagnosis, prediction of treatment outcome, and patient–treatment matching. Pain 24:143–158.

Index

Made in the USA
Monee, IL
07 July 2026